£1.50

General Practice Specialty Training

WITHDRAWN

Edited by Kay Mohanna and Abdol Tavabie

General Practice Specialty Training

Making it happen

**A practical guide for trainers, clinical
and educational supervisors**

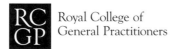

Royal College of
General Practitioners

The Royal College of General Practitioners was founded in 1952 with this object: *'To encourage, foster and maintain the highest possible standards in general practice and for that purpose to take or join with others in taking steps consistent with the charitable nature of that object which may assist towards the same.'*

Among its responsibilities under its Royal Charter the College is entitled to: *'Diffuse information on all matters affecting general practice and issue such publications as may assist the object of the College.'*

British Library Cataloguing-in-Publication Data
A catalogue record for this book is available from the British Library

© Royal College of General Practitioners, 2008
Published by the Royal College of General Practitioners, 2008
14 Princes Gate, Hyde Park, London SW7 1PU

All rights reserved. No part of this publication may be reproduced, stored in a retrieval system, or transmitted, in any form or by any means, electronic, mechanical, photocopying, recording or otherwise without the prior permission of the Royal College of General Practitioners.

DISCLAIMER
This publication is intended for the use of medical practitioners in the UK and not for patients. The authors, editors and publisher have taken care to ensure that the information contained in this book is correct to the best of their knowledge, at the time of publication. Whilst efforts have been made to ensure the accuracy of the information presented, particularly that related to the prescription of drugs, the authors, editors and publisher cannot accept liability for information that is subsequently shown to be wrong. Readers are advised to check that the information, especially that related to drug usage, complies with information contained in the *British National Formulary*, or equivalent, or manufacturers' datasheets, and that it complies with the latest legislation and standards of practice.

Designed and typeset at the Typographic Design Unit
Printed by Hobbs the Printers LTD
Indexed by Carol Ball

ISBN 978-0-85084-317-0

Contents

Foreword

With a brand new strategy for all medical specialty training, a new GP curriculum and a new assessment process, trainees, trainers and educational supervisors alike could be forgiven for being overtaken by the pace of change in general practice training. It was always the intention that there would be support materials for trainers and trainees, and this book is part of that support.

The curriculum clearly sets out the knowledge and competences required to become a general practitioner. *Being a General Practitioner*, the first curriculum statement, summarises the learning outcomes and is essential reading for anyone involved in specialty training for general practice. Familiarity with the nMRCGP is equally essential because it is now the required assessment for a Certificate of Completion of Training (CCT).

The curriculum reflects the breadth of general practice, something not previously attempted at national level. The nMRCGP indicates the need to demonstrate competence and incorporates a Clinical Skills Assessment, as well as more emphasis on performance in the workplace. Together these documents set out the academic base for the discipline of general practice. They were written primarily to meet the standards set by the Postgraduate Medical Education and Training Board (PMETB). To some, they may appear complex and challenging.

This book is different. The contributors were amongst those most involved in developing the curriculum and the assessment process – so they know their subjects well! Written with the needs of trainers in mind, it is full of practical advice about specialty training for general practice. It is intended for anyone involved in training for general practice – whether in hospital or in general practice. Trainers and educational supervisors have always played a significant role in supporting trainees; as a group they are keen to learn, keen to ensure high standards of training and keen to improve their own performance. This book will help.

We have entered a new era of training. All doctors wishing to enter general practice will now complete a planned programme of 'run-through training' and all must achieve the nMRCGP – the licence to practise. This gives a tremendous opportunity to reshape training for general practice, making it more appropriate to the needs of trainees and patients. This book is about making it happen.

Dr Bill Reith
Chair
RCGP POSTGRADUATE TRAINING BOARD
December 2007

Contributors

Dr Kay Mohanna is Vice-Chair of the RCGP Midlands Faculty and Associate Dean for GP assessment at the West Midlands Workforce Deanery. A trainer and co-facilitator for the West Midlands Modular Trainers course, she also runs 'teaching the teachers' courses for educational supervisors in the Foundation Programme and others in secondary care. Dr Mohanna is Principal Lecturer at Staffordshire University, where she is responsible for developing and delivering the MSc in Medical Education, and where she also teaches on healthcare ethics. Her chief interest is in faculty development and support for those involved in facilitating learning; her educational research has included work on evaluation of teaching practice and teaching styles. Dr Mohanna has co-authored nine books and edited two.

Prof. Abdol Tavabie is GP Dean and Deputy Dean Director at Kent, Surrey and Sussex Deanery. Prof. Tavabie has held various posts in GP education over the years including GP trainer, VTS course organiser, Associate GP Dean and Chairman of a Medical Audit Advisory Group. He has been GP Dean for Kent, Surrey and Sussex Deanery since 1998 and Vice-Chair of the Committee of General Practice Education Directors (COGPED). He is also Professor of Primary Care at the School of Health at the University of Brighton.

Contributing authors

☐ **Dr David Bruce**, Director of Postgraduate GP Education, Tayside Centre for General Practice (TCGP), Dundee.

☐ **Prof. Ruth Chambers**, GP and RCGP lead for Managed CPD and Essential General Practice.

☐ **Dr Nav Chana**, Associate Director of Postgraduate GP Education, London Deanery.

☐ **Dr Mark Coombe**, RCGP Wessex Faculty Director of Education, Deputy Convenor MRCGP consulting skills module.

☐ **Dr Mike Deighan**, Associate Dean, NHS West Midlands Workforce Deanery.

☐ **Dr Mei Ling Denney**, MRCGP Video Core Group member.

☐ **Prof. Steve Field**, Chair of Council, RCGP.

☐ **Dr Patti Gardiner**, Deputy Convenor Oral Core Group, MRCGP panel of examiners.

☐ **Dr Amar Rughani**, Associate Postgraduate Dean, South Yorkshire and South Humber Deanery, and RCGP assessor and Blueprinting clinical lead.

☐ **Joan Sargeant**, Associate Professor, Division of Medical Education, Dalhousie University, Halifax, Nova Scotia, Canada.

☐ **Dr Martin Wilkinson**, Head of Postgraduate School of General Practice and Acting Director of Postgraduate GP Education, NHS West Midlands Workforce Deanery.

x

Acknowledgements

This is a time of great change in general practice training, with an associated *xi* level of uncertainty and some apprehension felt by all those involved. So it has been a privilege to edit this book in an attempt to offer an outline of the process and some tips for success.

The pace of that change has been rapid and the book could not have been written without the expert input from others.

Chapter 3 draws heavily on earlier work by Tim Swanwick and Arthur Hibble, whose contributions are gratefully acknowledged.

The teaching styles questionnaire that appears in the Appendix is provided by the authors, Kay Mohanna, Ruth Chambers and David Wall, and with kind permission of the original publishers, Radcliffe.

Some of the content of Chapter 10 previously appeared in the published work-book accompanying the *Consulting: communication skills for GPs in training* DVD made by the Wessex Faculty of the RCGP, and is reproduced here with permission. General acknowledgements are also due to the Video Core Group of the RCGP, as well as members of the nMRCGP Workplace-Based Assessment (WPBA) Group for their help. Chapter 12 reproduces RCGP website information on the Applied Knowledge Test (AKT) written by the AKT core group.

In Chapter 13, the ECO feedback model was developed by Elaine McNaughton, David Bruce and Joan Sargeant. The two-question multi-source feedback (MSF) was developed by Douglas Murphy, David Bruce and Kevin Eva.

The work of Stewart Mercer in developing the CARE questionnaire is recognised as fundamental to the final WPBA tool described in Chapter 14.

Chapter 15 reproduces a list of online resources compiled by Luke Koupparis, with the kind permission of the author.

The RCGP would also like to acknowledge the support of the curriculum and assessment development teams, especially the ongoing work of Mike Deighan.

Dr Kay Mohanna
December 2007

Abbreviations

AAHE   American Association for Higher Education

ACGME   Accreditation Council for Graduate Medical Education

AED   automatic external defibrillator

AKT   Applied Knowledge Test

ARCP   annual review of competence progression

BMA   British Medical Association

BMJ   *British Medical Journal*

CARE   Consultation and Relational Empathy measure

CbD   case-based discussion

CCT   Certificate of Completion of Training

COGPED Committee of General Practice Education Directors

COPMeD Conference of Postgraduate Medical Deans

COT   consultation observation tool

CPD   continuous professional development

CPR   current cardiopulmonary resuscitation

CSA   Clinical Skills Assessment

CSR   Clinical Supervisor's Report

DISQ   Doctors' Interpersonal Skills Questionnaire

DOPS   direct observation of procedural skills

EBHC   evidence-based health care

EMQ   extending matching questions

ETR   Enhanced Trainer's Report

FT   Foundation Programme training

GMC   General Medical Council

GPAQ   General Practice Assessment Questionnaire

GPStR   GP specialty registrar

GPwSI   GP with a Special Interest

HES   Hospital Episode Statistics

IAEA   International Association for Educational Assessment

LMC   Local Medical Committee

MCQ   multiple-choice question

mini-CEX mini-clinical evaluation exercise

MMC   *Modernising Medical Careers*

MMR   measles, mumps and rubella immunisation

MSF   multi-source feedback

NICE   National Institute for Health and Clinical Excellence

OOH   out of hours

OSCE   objective structured clinical examination

PCT	Primary Care Trust
PDP	Personal Development Plan
PHCT	Primary Health Care Team
PMETB	Postgraduate Medical Education and Training Board
PSA	prostate-specific antigen
PSGP	Postgraduate School of General Practice
PSQ	patient satisfaction questionnaire
QA	quality assurance
QM	quality management
QOF	Quality and Outcomes Framework
RCP	Royal College of Physicians
RCGP	Royal College of General Practitioners
SBA	single best answer
SD	standard deviation
SEA	significant event analysis
SHEFFPAT	Sheffield Patient Assessment Tool
SHO	Senior House Officer
SMART	Specific, Measurable, Attainable, Relevant, Time-signalled
SOLO	Structure of Observed Learning Outcomes
STA	Specialist Training Authority of the Medical Royal Colleges
WPBA	Workplace-Based Assessment

1 Overview of GP specialty training

Developing the modern generalist for the community setting

Abdol Tavabie

This book seeks to introduce and explain the new training and assessment process for general practice. In this chapter we look at the history and rationale for developing the new general practice (GP) specialty training programmes. We also cover the role and responsibilities of individuals and organisations in preparing the future community generalists for their work in the NHS.

The career pathway of doctors in all specialties, after qualifying at medical school, is underpinned by the professional values described by the General Medical Council in *Good Medical Practice*[1] and a commitment to improving the quality and safety of patient care through structured training programmes. Two key strategy documents, *Unfinished Business*[2] and *Modernising Medical Careers*,[3] have informed the revision of postgraduate medical training.

Modernising Medical Careers (MMC) marks a major reform in postgraduate medical education. It aims to improve patient care by delivering a focused career structure for doctors. Securing quality of care and patient safety is at the heart of the reform. It offers postgraduate medical trainees the chance to gain insight into possible career options or to build a wider appreciation of medicine before embarking on specialist training (also known as 'run through training').

MMC was developed initially from the need to reform the Senior House Officer (SHO) grade that was identified in *Unfinished Business*. Previously half of all SHO appointments were short term and only one third of GPs had completed formal GP vocational training programmes. MMC also recognised and responded to changes in working patterns following introduction of new working time regulations.[4] An underlying principle was to deliver all postgraduate training within managed, competence-assessed training programmes with clear curricula and assessment tools.

BOX 1.1 The role and responsibility of MMC

MMC was established in 2003 as a Department of Health project with the aim of making changes to delivery of medical education and training. MMC is a non-statutory body, accountable to the four Departments of Health (for England, Scotland, Wales and Northern Ireland). It is charged to determine the career pathways for postgraduate medical education and has developed four separate strands of programmes, including process of recruitment and selection to specialty training programmes.

Implementation of MMC was in two stages.

Stage 1 was implemented in August 2005. This consists of the two-year foundation programmes that require postgraduate doctors to demonstrate abilities and competence against set standards.[5] The foundation programme follows on from medical school graduation and develops doctors to be more able to recognise learning opportunities and take advantage of them within a framework of competence-based assessment. This uses workplace-based assessment against clearly defined learning outcomes.

Stage 2 commenced in August 2007. This is specialist training (run through training) as managed, competence-based programmes.[6]

The new specialty training for general practice programme is a minimum of three years' duration, after completing the foundation programme, and should ideally:

- be broad and balanced
- be based in general practice
- provide the GP trainee with managed exposure to a range of relevant and appropriate specialist disciplines.

BOX 1.2 **Ensuring a balanced training programme**

Stop here, and consider how you would ensure that every GP specialty registrar (GPStR) has a broad, balanced training programme, if you were in charge.

Consider how you would achieve an appropriate balance between a GPStR's clinical and learning experience to run the service and meet the required learning outcomes.

A key driver for change in the quality management of postgraduate medical education has been the establishment of the Postgraduate Medical Education and Training Board (PMETB).[7] PMETB is an independent statutory body, accountable to Parliament, responsible for overseeing and promoting the development of postgraduate medical education for all specialties, including general practice. It was established by the General and Specialist Medical Practice (Education, Training and Qualifications) Order 2003, and approved by Parliament on 4 April 2003 to develop a single, unifying framework for postgraduate medical education.

Several reports – including those from the working group on specialist medical training,[8] *The NHS Plan*,[9] and the Bristol Inquiry[10] – indicated a need to establish such an independent overarching regulator of postgraduate medical training, with due public and NHS representations and influence. In addition, *Unfinished Business* also concluded by identifying a need for an independent training board to ensure that, throughout training, all assessments are appropriate, valid and reliable with defined learning outcomes to demonstrate achievement of independent practitioner status.

There has been a good deal of confusion about the roles of PMETB and MMC, as they were established at much the same time. MMC is the UK strategy initiative and PMETB is the UK competent authority discharging functions required under European Community law.[11] It is accountable to Parliament and determines standards of postgraduate medical education in the UK.

BOX 1.3 The role and responsibility of PMETB

- To define standards of, and requirements relating to, postgraduate medical education and training.
- To ensure the maintenance of the established standards and requirements.
- To develop and promote postgraduate medical education and training in the UK.

3

Box 1.4 summarises the activities of PMETB since it was formed in 2005.

BOX 1.4 Activities of the PMETB

- Working with medical royal colleges to approve the curricula of all medical specialties.
- Approving assessment methodology against PMETB's principles.
- Initiating national surveys of doctors in training. It is compulsory for all trainees to take part in surveys that measure trainees' perceptions of their training provider's compliance with the PMETB generic standards for training.[12]
- Surveying clinical and educational supervisors who are involved with training of specialty trainees to measure their readiness as well as their organisation in training programmes.
- Quality management of training programmes to ensure that its standards for training are being met by deaneries across the UK.
- Developing a 'triggered visits' process to enable them to respond to concerns of serious educational failure needing prompt investigation.
- Issuing Certificates of Completion of Training (CCT) to those doctors who successfully complete postgraduate training prospectively approved, in collaboration with medical royal colleges.
- Establishing equivalence routes to specialist registration for those doctors who have not followed a traditional training programme, but who may have gained the same level of skills and knowledge as CCT holders.[13]

New GP specialty training programme

In the case of general practice PMETB recognised that the new GP specialty training needed:[14]

- an appropriate curriculum defining intended learning outcomes relevant to the role of a generalist in the community setting
- GPStRs to be able to develop a range of appropriate generic skills and attitudes
- a learner-centred approach to educational programmes

- an appropriate level of supervision of GP specialty trainees with regular constructive feedback
- GPStRs to continue to develop their knowledge and skills, and to adapt to changes in healthcare delivery
- a competence-based approach to assessment underpinned by rigorous assessment tools demonstrating the appropriate learning outcomes
- clear sets of quality standards relating to all aspects of the delivery of medical education including quality of learning environments, quality of teaching and assessment, and documentation of all evidence collected by GP specialty trainees and their supervisors.

BOX 1.5 Achieving learner-centred education

Stop and think.

What does learner-centred education mean and how would you achieve it? What are the benefits of this approach to learner and service?

What are the implications of this approach for the responsibilities of the learners for their own learning, and for you in your capacity?

Delivering the GP specialty training curriculum

The design of the GP curriculum marks a watershed in postgraduate training for general practice. It is the first national GP training curriculum and offers a unique opportunity to shape GP training to be fit for purpose for working in the NHS. It is designed to highlight a range of knowledge, competences and clinical attitudes considered necessary for a generalist in independent practice. The work of GPs has been a fundamental part of healthcare services in the UK since inception of the National Health Service in 1948. The importance of general practitioners as generalists has been emphasised by changes to the structure of the NHS, such as the development of the *Primary Care Led NHS*,[15] *Our Health, Our Care, Our Say*[16] and the emergence of Primary Care Trusts (PCTs) as major commissioners of health care for local populations across the UK.[17]

One criticism of a competence-based curriculum is that in attempting to describe competences and meet learning outcomes, it constrains the learner.[18] The GP curriculum avoids this criticism by defining both generic competences and specific learning outcomes across the breadth of general practice. The curriculum is designed to be delivered over the duration of the specialty training programme. During hospital placements, GPStRs will be working towards general practice-based learning outcomes relevant to the specialty in which they are working, as well as looking to develop the more generic competences.

PMETB has set standards relating to the type and balance of experience that a GPStR needs to have achieved when applying for a CCT. These were based on recommendations from the Royal College of General Practitioners (RCGP).

4

GP postgraduate schools (see also Chapter 5) are responsible for ensuring that the GP curriculum is being delivered in hospital posts and that individual programmes for GPStRs are sufficiently balanced to meet CCT requirements.

GP specialty training is built around three-year programmes, which involve a series of placements lasting a minimum of 12 months in a hospital setting and at least 12 months in general practice. However, the RCGP has stated that ideally a minimum of 18 months will be required for GPStRs to gain general practice competences in the community. Selection into GP specialty training is based on meeting the GP person specification (available from www.gprecruitment.org.uk/vacancies/specification.htm). Those trainees wishing to enter GP specialty training on completion of the foundation programme will enter at Specialty Registrar Year One (ST1); those trainees with one year's experience and training in SHO posts will enter a training programme at Specialty Registrar Year Two (ST2); those who have already undertaken a minimum of two years' SHO posts relevant to general practice training will enter to Specialty Registrar Year Three (ST3). A person specification for each stage exists and entry is subject to demonstrating eligibility. (More detail is available on the National GP Recruitment Office website.)

Effective delivery of the GP curriculum requires changes to existing patterns of working and training provision. There are summarised in Box 1.6.

BOX 1.6 Principles of GP specialty training

- Each GPStR must have a designated educational supervisor who will be a GP, to oversee and review his or her progress every six months.

- Educational and clinical supervisors need to have a shared understanding in primary and secondary care of the core GP competences, to provide an integrated programme for each GPStR.

- All placements need to allow GPStRs the opportunity to develop appropriate GP competences.

- Educational events in hospital departments and primary care need to reflect the learning outcomes of the GP curriculum.

- Training for hospital clinical supervisors will be required and ideally this should include joint learning with GPs in order to increase shared understanding.

- Training programmes for GP trainers will need to reflect the new curriculum and assessment processes.

- GPStRs will need support in understanding how to use the curriculum and to recognise the breadth of learning opportunities that can be accessed in hospital and GP placements.

- GP educators will need to be trained in group dynamics, small-group facilitation skills and educational management.

5

Assessment

PMETB has also laid down principles and standards for assessments in specialty training. The Workplace-Based Assessment (WPBA) methodology developed for general practice is formative in approach and uses tools congruent with those in the foundation programme that facilitate regular feedback.[19] The challenge has been to develop tools that not only demonstrate what a doctor 'can do'[20] in ideal circumstances but can also be used to look at how they actually perform in the reality of everyday clinical practice.[21] Chapter 7 describes good practice in assessment and how the e-portfolio will facilitate coordination between postgraduate schools, GPStRs and the RCGP.

An additional challenge is to ensure GPStRs and clinical supervisors recognise and make the most of these assessment processes as learning opportunities. Clinical and educational supervisors need to be trained in undertaking assessments as recommended in *A Guide to Postgraduate Specialty Training in the UK* ('The Gold Guide').[22]

BOX 1.7 **Opportunities for collaborative working**

Stop and think.

The new GP specialty training offers the opportunity to work and learn with your colleagues across primary and secondary care. What is your experience so far, and how can it be improved for the benefit of patients and GPStRs?

What are the opportunities for collaborative working focused on teaching, and how can this be facilitated?

The CCT application process

The RCGP, working with the PMETB, took on a more direct role in evaluating specialty training for general practice in 2005. All GPStRs must register with the RCGP at the beginning of their training programme. Not only will this trigger access to a personal e-portfolio to record all learning activities, assessment and feedback but will also ensure that the RCGP is informed of the outcome of the annual review of competence progression (ARCP). This annual review is a postgraduate school-level activity where the training of each GPStR is monitored to ensure satisfactory progress (see Chapter 5). The RCGP is thus the body that monitors training nationally to ensure that each GPStR achieves the level of competence required for independent practice.

At the end of the training period, there are two routes to the award of a CCT.

Article 10 of the postgraduate training regulations for general practice applies to those undergoing standard training within a programme approved in advance by PMETB. This will apply to the vast majority of GPStRs. For every GPStR, the RCGP Certification Unit will receive the outcome of the final ARCP directly from his or her postgraduate school. In addition, towards the end of training, GPStRs will obtain a PMETB application form from the RCGP Certification Unit. On completion this form must be sent directly to PMETB with the required fee and supporting documents to apply for the CCT. The RCGP will check all Article 10 trainees and, following RCGP recommendation, the PMETB will issue a CCT when the GPStR's application is received.

Article 11 applies when a non-standard training programme has been followed to meet the requirements for entry to the specialist register through an equivalent route. This might be because the GPStR has asked for training overseas to be taken into account, or when the training programme has not had prior PMETB approval because, for example, a new post was incorporated. In this case PMETB will first need to approve the training programme. Again, the RCGP is responsible for ensuring satisfactory competence of the GPStR depending on the outcome of the final ARCP. On receipt of the trainee's application form, PMETB will issue a CCT only if both the training programme meets the required standards for breadth and depth of training and the RCGP confirms the competence of the GPStR.

If PMETB decides that a GPStR is not eligible for a certificate this will be communicated to him or her, in writing, with reasons. If further training might help, recommendation for this will be made. (Further and the most up-to-date information can be found on the RCGP website at www.rcgp.org.uk.)

The role and responsibility of the RCGP

The RCGP has an important duty under the law to ensure that GPStRs who are awarded the CCT are fit for independent practice as GPs.

- All medical royal colleges (including the RCGP) are responsible for determining the specialty curricula and submitting them for consideration by the PMETB.
- RCGP will work closely with postgraduate deaneries to ensure that the GP curriculum is being fully implemented.
- The RCGP will provide national supervision of GP training to ensure consistent, equitable standards throughout the UK.
- The RCGP will work closely with heads of GP schools and the Committee of General Practice Education Directors (COGPED) in setting and monitoring the standards of WPBAs to ensure that there is consistency across deaneries.
- Membership of the RCGP has been designed as the licensing process to assess GPStRs who have undertaken the UK's GP specialty training programme in preparation of a CCT.
- The RCGP is implementing two of three components of the MRCGP (the applied knowledge test [AKT] and the clinical skills assessment [CSA]) nationally (see Chapter 2).
- The RCGP is responsible for assessment of GPStRs and makes the recommendation to the PMETB for CCT certification.

- The RCGP has a role in supporting education by giving advice to trainees, and supporting educational supervisors.
- The RCGP will take part in the deaneries' ARCP panels to monitor performance of GPStRs and collect information and data nationally.

8   The role of postgraduate deanery and GP schools

Postgraduate deaneries are responsible for the organisation and quality management of postgraduate medical education, and are expected to work with medical royal colleges. They are accountable to the PMETB for their educational management activities. Postgraduate deaneries are responsible for:

- overseeing the systems and process to commission postgraduate medical training from educational providers (hospital trusts, GP practices and others)
- setting up GP schools or comparable committees to manage GP specialty training programmes (Chapter 5 will describe fully the organisational structure and functions of GP schools)
- recruitment and selection based on national process and guidance
- developing appropriate systems to ensure that GP curricula are being implemented effectively
- the development of faculties of clinical teachers and monitoring their activities
- setting up quality management systems, and quality control learning environment, teaching and assessment methodology
- setting up the ARCP panels and monitoring their activities.

BOX 1.8 Implementing change

Stop and consider the following in your organisation.
- Who are currently the key personnel involved in GP training?
- How is the quality of educational provision managed and evaluated?
- What are the barriers to implementing change?
- How can you influence change?

The Role of GP programme directors

GP programme directors are tasked to oversee delivery of the GP curriculum in both hospital and general practice placements locally, and work with clinical and educational supervisors to coordinate appropriate feedback, assessment, handover and (if required) delivery of educational programmes for GPStRs. GP programme directors will act as a conduit between GPStRs, clinical and educational supervisors and deanery to ensure the smooth delivery of GP curriculum and assessments. The following are examples of their activities:

- overseeing delivery of the local GP specialty training of the GPStRs in their programme
- coordinating GPStRs' induction programmes
- coordinating matching educational supervisor and GPStRs
- overseeing delivery of GP curriculum and assessment in hospital posts
- overseeing delivery of educational programmes for GPStRs
- facilitating meaningful handover processes.

9

This chapter has outlined the background to, and structure of, GP specialty training. Key to success, however, will be the attitude of the individual GPStRs, who are expected to take an active role in their own learning. GPStRs should make it their responsibility to establish what is expected of them and ensure they play an active and professional role in the healthcare team involved in patient care. They should ensure that they fulfil their contractual duties about hours of work, but not work beyond these hours and potentially put patient safety at risk. They must ensure that they do not work beyond their capability or spend excess time on tasks with little educational benefit. They must find the balance between service and educational commitments. They should be supported to become mature, reflective practitioners able to identify and respond to their own learning needs.

Educational opportunities will be provided and quality assured within the postgraduate schools following the changes under MMC and in accordance with the standards set by the PMETB. However, GPStRs are expected to ensure that they carry out a mix of clinical, managerial and educational responsibilities. They will demonstrate commitment to the GP programme and ensure that they complete any preparation for teaching, and group tasks. The following are some of the more important activities:

- securing the safety of patients and seek help when appropriate
- demonstrating active involvement in team working
- seeking constructive feedback, and reflecting and acting appropriately upon it
- being registered with the RCGP to have access to e-portfolio
- establishing methods of regular communication with clinical and educational supervisors
- planning and discussing their learning, assessments and periodic review with their clinical and educational supervisors
- taking part in the PMETB trainees' survey
- leading on their own required assessments
- undertaking assessments at the appropriate time
- taking an active role in clinical and group discussions.

REFERENCES

1. General Medical Council. *Good Medical Practice* (third edn) London: GMC, 2001.

2. Donaldson L. *Unfinished Business* London: DH, 2002.

3. Department of Health. *Modernising Medical Careers: the next steps* London: DH, 2004.

4. European Union Directives. *The Working Time Directive*, 93/104/EC November 1993

5. Department of Health. *A Guide to Foundation Training* London: DH, 2005.

6. Department of Health. *Career Management: an approach for medical schools, deaneries, royal colleges and trusts* London: The Stationery Office, 2005.

7. Postgraduate Medical Education and Training Board. *Strategy Document 2006–2010* London: PMETB, 2005.

8. Department of Health. *Hospital Doctors: training for the future. The report of the working group on specialist medical training* London: DH, 2003.

9. Department of Health. *The NHS Plan: a plan for investment, a plan for reform* London: DH, 2000.

10. The Stationery Office. *The Bristol Royal Infirmary Inquiry Final Report* London: HMSO, 2001.

11. The European Specialist Medical Qualifications Order Statutory Instrument No. 3208, 1995.

12. Postgraduate Medical Education and Training Board. *Generic Standards for Training* London: PMETB, 2006.

13. Postgraduate Medical Education and Training Board. *General Guidance on Evidence to Submit with Application under Article 11* London: PMETB, 2005.

14. Royal College of General Practitioners. RCGP curriculum website, www.rcgp-curriculum.org.uk [accessed December 2007].

15. Department of Health. *Primary Care Led NHS* London: DH, 2004.

16. Department of Health. *Our Health, Our Care, Our Say: a new direction for community services* London: DH, 2007.

17. Department of Health. *Primary Care Trust: Commissioner of Health* London: DH, 2004.

18. Talbot M. Monkey see, monkey do: a critique of the competency model in graduate medical education *Medical Education* 2004; 38: 587–92.

19. Swanwick T, Chana N. Workplace assessment for licensing in general practice *British Journal of General Practice* 2005; 55(515): 461–7.

20. Miller GE. The assessment of clinical skills/competence/performance *Academic Medicine* 1990; 65: 563–7.

21. Rethens J-J, Sturmans F, Drop R, *et al.* The relationship between competence and performance: implications for assessing practice performance *Medical Education* 2001; 36: 901–9.

22. Department of Health. *A Guide to Postgraduate Specialty Training in the UK: the gold guide* London: DH, 2007, www.mmc.nhs.uk/download_files/Gold_Guide_290607.doc [accessed December 2007].

2 Assessment in general practice training

Steve Field

Introduction

The new general practice curriculum was granted unconditional approval by the Postgraduate Medical Education and Training Board (PMETB) in 2006. The important part of the curriculum dealing with assessment of the trainee, provisionally called the nMRCGP, was approved by the PMETB in early 2007. The curriculum as a whole went 'live' across the UK on 1 August 2007. Once the transition period is over, this assessment package will be known simply as MRCGP.

The curriculum is the first nationally approved curriculum for training general practitioners. It provides a new system for education, training and assessment, replacing both the outdated Vocational Training Regulations and the dual-assessment system of summative assessment as the licensing examination and the old College examination.

The curriculum is designed as a guide for the period of postgraduate medical education for general practice from the end of the Foundation Programme to completion of specialist training. Those who successfully complete their training and achieve the required standard in their assessments will be awarded the PMETB's Certificate of Completion of Training (CCT), which in turn gives the successful doctor eligibility for entry onto the General Medical Council's (GMC) General Practitioner Register.

This chapter gives an overview of the development of the new curriculum and an outline of the GP assessment package.

Development of the curriculum

The curriculum work began in 2001. The RCGP's Education Network established two working groups, one to deal with teaching and learning, and the other with assessment. Each group brought together experts in education, training and assessment, from the College, from deaneries and from universities across the UK. They included patient, public and GP trainee representation as well as management input from the NHS.

A literature review was commissioned from the Centre for Research into Medical and Dental Education at the University of Birmingham and an extensive consultation exercise was carried out. This involved a national question-naire survey of the views of trainees and GP educators on training for general practice, meetings with lay representatives and GP trainees, and focus groups and presentations at national and international conferences to share findings and explore perspectives on them.

Following the consultation period the core curriculum statement, *Being a General Practitioner*, was written, together with more detailed supplementary statements. The statements were circulated widely in draft form to more stake-holders, lay and trainee representatives as well as specialist interest groups within the RCGP, and posted on the RCGP website. There followed a further period of even wider formal consultation prior to submission of the curriculum to the PMETB for approval. It was approved unconditionally in 2006, a testi-mony to the hard work and extensive consultation exercise.

The curriculum specifies a framework for a structured educational pro-gramme to address the knowledge, competences, clinical and communication skills, and professional attitudes considered appropriate for a doctor intending to undertake practice in the contemporary UK National Health Service. The framework draws explicitly upon *The European Definition of General Practice/Family Medicine* as set out by the European Academy of Teachers in General Practice (EURACT)[1] and has been mapped against *Good Medical Practice*, the GMC's guidance on the duties of a doctor registered with the GMC.[2]

The *European Definition of General Practice/Family Medicine* contains six domains of core competence described on a background of three essential features fundamental to a person-centred scientific discipline. From these the RCGP developed generic competences of the general practitioner, and also subject-specific competences.

These six domains of competence are:

1 ◊ primary care management
2 ◊ person-centred care
3 ◊ specific problem-solving skills
4 ◊ a comprehensive approach
5 ◊ community orientation
6 ◊ a holistic approach.

The three essential features fundamental to a person-centred scientific disci-pline are:

1 ◊ CONTEXTUAL – using the context of the person, the family, the community and his or her culture
2 ◊ ATTITUDINAL – based on the doctor's professional capabilities, values and ethics
3 ◊ SCIENTIFIC – adopting a critical and research-based approach to practice and maintaining this through continuing learning and quality improvement.

The framework is set within a pedagogical approach that supports the preparation of lifelong learners. This is a necessary prerequisite for doctors to sustain their capacity to practise effectively in an environment of changing expectations about appropriate practice. It is an approach that also recognises that individuals learn at different rates using different styles and, typically, that learning is enhanced when individuals are actively involved in identifying their needs and contribute to planning, implementing and evaluating their programme of learning.

The curriculum has been developed with three principal audiences in mind: trainees, educators and assessors. For trainees, it contains the elements of knowledge, skills and attitudes that will assist them in reaching and demonstrating required competences. For educators with responsibilities as facilitators or managers of learning, it is a framework that, shaped by professional practice, is a basis for their dialogues with trainees as learners. For assessors, it is a resource that enables them to interpret learning outcomes into valid and reliable tests of those competences.

Development of the nMRCGP

In the past, trainees were subjected to two assessment systems: the licensing assessment called summative assessment, which everyone had to pass, and the MRCGP examination, set at a higher standard, which was optional.

The MRCGP examination began in 1965. Since then, there has been a process of continual evolution as the discipline of general practice itself has evolved and as assessment methodologies have developed. It was widely acclaimed in the UK and across the world.

The final configuration of the old MRCGP involved a multiple-choice test, a written examination, an oral examination and a test of consulting skills (either an assessment of the doctor's own videotaped consultations or a simulated surgery). While it became compulsory for membership of the College in 1968, it was not compulsory for entry into the profession, although the vast majority sat and passed the MRCGP as a demonstration that they had achieved the optimal standard for general practitioners.

Summative assessment was introduced for all GP registrars completing their training in September 1996. Its controversial introduction was one of the biggest changes in vocational training for general practice. There was evidence that the existing informal assessment of trainees by their trainers was not rigorous enough to weed out incompetent trainees.[3] The public wanted reassurance that only doctors who had achieved an agreed minimum standard of competence would be able to enter the profession. Summative assessment tested minimal competence in a wide range of knowledge, skills and attitudes required of an independent general practitioner. Whilst a very few incompetent doctors were identified by the system, the vast majority of GP registrars had no difficulty in passing summative assessment. The term 'minimal competence' was felt to be

13

demeaning by many trainees and their trainers. Increasing numbers, therefore, took the MRCGP examination to prove that they had reached the optimum (often called 'gold standard') rather than the minimum standard.

Summative assessment had four key components: an audit project; an assessment of videotaped consultations; a test of factual knowledge; and the structured trainer's report. The GP trainer completed this report during the course of the trainee's year in general practice, to document that the trainee had demonstrated the core skills required to be a competent GP.

All trainees had to successfully complete the structured trainer's report, but trainees who wished to gain membership to the College often sat the two different multiple-choice question (MCQ) tests and submitted two different videotapes for assessment. As more doctors opted to take the MRCGP, the assessments grew closer together, with a single route to assessment of the videotaped consultations helping to reduce the burden of assessment on trainees and their trainers. The feedback from trainees and their trainers demonstrated their irritation with the two different systems. It was obvious that neither the summative assessment system nor the old MRCGP were fit for purpose. Neither met the requirements of PMETB, nor would they meet the RCGP's needs to assess trainees pursuing the new curriculum. The situation was untenable and confusing.

It was from this base that the assessment working group began, in partnership with those working on the curriculum as a whole. Each of the new assessment tools was chosen on the basis of best practice. The working group ensured that decisions were based on rational arguments and referenced to contemporary psychometric and educational evidence. It developed an overarching and coherent strategy relating to the entire training period, which encourages progression and future professional development.

The new assessment system, called the nMRCGP, was approved by the PMETB in 2007. After cessation of the current examination in 2008 it will be known simply as the MRCGP.

The nMRCGP

The new assessment system is delivered by the RCGP in partnership with the postgraduate deaneries across the UK. It is a combination of Workplace-Based Assessments intended to cover the whole three years of training and two nationally delivered assessments.

The three components are:

1 ◊ the APPLIED KNOWLEDGE TEST ◊ a multiple-choice question paper
2 ◊ the CLINICAL SKILLS ASSESSMENT ◊ an objective structured clinical examination (OSCE)-style skills assessment
3 ◊ the WORKPLACE-BASED ASSESSMENT ◊ a continuous assessment based on an Enhanced Trainer's Report (ETR).

The Applied Knowledge Test

The RCGP describes the Applied Knowledge Test (AKT) as 'a summative assessment of the knowledge base that underpins independent general practice in the United Kingdom within the context of the National Health Service. Candidates who pass this assessment will have demonstrated their competence in applying knowledge at a level which is sufficiently high for independent practice.'[4]

GPStR registrars may attempt the AKT at any point during their time in training. However, the highest chance of success is likely to be when they are in the final year of their specialty training programme. A pass 'expires' if the rest of nMRCGP is not completed within three years of the AKT, which will then need to be taken again.

The test is a three-hour multiple-choice question paper consisting of 200 items of single best answer and extended matching questions. It is computer based and delivered at 150 professional testing centres around the UK.

It tests both clinical and non-clinical aspects of general practice knowledge and assesses the application of knowledge, including decision making, evaluation of evidence and undifferentiated problems, and decisions regarding patient safety.

The questions in the AKT are based on the knowledge contained within the RCGP curriculum, distributed as follows:

- clinical medicine (80 per cent)
- health informatics and administrative issues (10 per cent)
- critical appraisal and evidence-based clinical practice (10 per cent).

The Clinical Skills Assessment

The RCGP describes the CSA as 'an assessment of a doctor's ability to integrate and apply clinical, professional, communication and practical skills appropriate for general practice'.[5] GPStRs are eligible to take the CSA when they are within 12 months of the expected date of completing their training.

This form of assessment will be familiar to most candidates because it is similar to the OSCE used in UK medical schools.

Each candidate is allocated a room set up as a GP consulting room with very basic medical kit provided. The candidates are expected to bring their own equipment with them (the RCGP describes this as the 'equipment generally found in a doctor's bag'). The RCGP will specify exactly what is needed with confirmation of candidates' applications to take the assessment – keep an eye on the website at www.rcgp.org.uk/the_gp_journey/nmrcgp.aspx.

The candidates remain in their allotted consulting room throughout the CSA. Each CSA consists of 13 consultations, each of ten minutes' duration; 12 are assessed, with one consultation being used for piloting scenarios for future examinations. At the start of the assessment a buzzer will sound, and the first 'patient' will knock on the candidate's door. At the end of 10 minutes, another buzzer will sound, and the 'patient' will leave the room. After a short break of two minutes, the next case begins with the sounding of the next buzzer. This process is repeated until all 13 cases have been seen.

The patients are played by professional role-players, trained and calibrated so that they can perform their role in a consistent manner. The cases are marked by trained and calibrated MRCGP assessors. They mark the same case all day, to ensure reliability.

The assessors follow the 'patient' into the consulting room and mark the case as it unfolds, sitting out of the candidate's line of view. They do not interact with the candidate unless required to do so. This may occur, for example, if the candidate wants to examine the patient in a way that is unnecessary for the case marking, requests a piece of information that the role-player cannot provide, or indicates that he or she would normally use a particular piece of clinical equipment. Most of the time, they will just observe the doctor–patient consultation and remain silent.

The CSA has been designed to test mainly the following areas of the curriculum:

- PRIMARY CARE MANAGEMENT ◊ recognition and management of common medical conditions in primary care
- PROBLEM-SOLVING SKILLS ◊ gathering and using data for clinical judgement, choice of examination, investigations and their interpretation. Demonstration of a structured and flexible approach to decision making
- COMPREHENSIVE APPROACH ◊ demonstration of proficiency in the management of co-morbidity and risk
- PERSON-CENTRED CARE ◊ communication with patient and the use of recognised consultation techniques to promote a shared approach to managing problems
- ATTITUDINAL ASPECTS ◊ practising ethically with respect for equality and diversity, with accepted professional codes of conduct
- CLINICAL PRACTICAL SKILLS ◊ demonstrating proficiency in performing physical examinations and using diagnostic/therapeutic instruments.

The consultations used in the CSA are called 'cases'. A great amount of time and energy has gone into writing the cases by very experienced GPs who have had training in case writing. All of the cases relate to the new curriculum and are informed by real consultations that the case writers have experienced themselves. This ensures that they are representative of current general practice in the UK. The consultations will, therefore, include male and female patients, children, adults and the elderly. The case mix will include acute and chronic illness, undifferentiated presentations, health promotion issues, and consultations with patients who have psychological or social problems.

Candidates are given written mock medical case notes. The medical case notes will contain information including any relevant past medical history, current medication, social habits, etc. Previous consultations might also be provided, or a relevant letter from a hospital consultant, a set of blood test results or even an ECG. The assessors and the role-players are briefed in advance and supplied with more detailed information.

The type of consultations that a candidate might expect to encounter will reflect what happens in any GP's surgery in the UK, e.g. communicating sensitively with a depressed patient and assessing his or her suicide risk, checking and demonstrating the inhaler technique of a patient with asthma, consulting with someone who is 'tired all the time' or discussing the treatment options with a hypertensive patient.

Each consultation is assessed separately by making judgements in three broad areas (the assessors call these 'domains'). These are: information gathering; clinical management; and interpersonal skills. The performance for each consultation is then graded as Clear Pass, Marginal Pass, Marginal Fail or Clear Fail. The candidate must pass a certain number of cases to pass the assessment overall. The exact number is the subject of ongoing standard-setting exercises.

The Workplace-Based Assessment

The RCGP places great importance on trainees learning and being assessed in their workplace. It describes WPBA for nMRCGP as 'the evaluation of a doctor's progress in their performance over time, in those areas of professional practice best tested in the workplace'.[6] WPBA should not be thought of as a series of pass–fail assessments. It is an opportunity for gathering evidence of how the GPStR is performing and giving feedback on that performance.

The WPBA is designed to integrate teaching, learning and assessment. It is the opportunity for the assessment process to get close to the real situations in which GPs work. It enables assessment of some areas of competence that are hard to disentangle from system (e.g. practice facilities) or personal influences (e.g. health). These include areas of professionalism including probity, time keeping and team working.

Trainees should know what is expected of them and have an opportunity to demonstrate attainment over time and in a variety of contexts. The WPBAs are designed to provide the trainee with feedback on their strengths and areas that need development. It will also drive learning in important areas of competence and determine whether the trainee is ready to progress to the next stage of their career. It will, of course, identify those trainees in difficulty during their training so that appropriate support may be offered by the deanery.

The WPBA is designed around the ETR, and the individual assessments, reflections and learning are recorded in the e-portfolio. The evidence will enable their trainer to judge and provide feedback on their progress in 12 designated MRCGP assessment domains, which are derived from the core curriculum statement, *Being a General Practitioner.*

The 12 nMRCGP assessment domains

1 ☐ COMMUNICATION AND CONSULTATION SKILLS

This includes how a GP communicates with patients and uses recognised consultation models and communication techniques.

2 ☐ PRACTISING HOLISTICALLY

This considers the ability of the doctor to operate in physical, psychological, socioeconomic and cultural dimensions, taking into account feelings as well as thoughts.

3 ☐ DATA GATHERING AND INTERPRETATION

This involves the gathering and use of data for making clinical judgements, the choice of physical examinations and investigations, and how they are interpreted.

4 ☐ MAKING A DIAGNOSIS/MAKING DECISIONS

This examines how a GP adopts a structured, conscious approach to decision making.

5 ☐ CLINICAL MANAGEMENT

This assesses how a doctor recognises and manages common medical conditions in primary care.

6 ☐ MANAGING MEDICAL COMPLEXITY AND PROMOTING HEALTH

This looks at the aspects of care that go beyond managing straightforward problems, including the management of co-morbidity, uncertainty, risk and approaches to health rather than just illness.

7 ☐ PRIMARY CARE ADMINISTRATION AND IMT

This includes the appropriate use of primary care administration systems, effective record keeping and information technology for the benefit of patient care.

8 ☐ WORKING WITH COLLEAGUES AND IN TEAMS

GPs must be able to work effectively with other health professionals to ensure good patient care, including the sharing of information with colleagues.

9 ☐ COMMUNITY ORIENTATION

This involves managing the health and social care of the practice population and local community.

10 ☐ MAINTAINING PERFORMANCE, LEARNING AND TEACHING

This looks at how doctors maintain their performance and ensure effective continuing professional development of themselves and others.

11 ☐ MAINTAINING AN ETHICAL APPROACH TO PRACTICE

This examines how GPs ensure they practise ethically, with integrity and a respect for diversity.

12 ☐ FITNESS TO PRACTISE

This involves the GP's awareness of when his or her own performance, conduct or health, or that of others, might put patients at risk and the actions taken to protect patients.

The WPBA also includes assessment of the trainees' important psychomotor skills, i.e. the clinical and practical skills specific to general practice.

Most of the evidence that GPStRs collect will be 'naturally occurring'. It will be gathered informally or by using specially designed assessment tools. The evidence will be recorded in their e-portfolio throughout their three-year training programme, in hospital and in general practice settings. At the six-month reviews conducted by the educational supervisor or trainer, it will be used to inform the decision made about their progress.

Because the WPBA is not pass/fail, there is no pass/fail standard to any of the assessment tools. The tools are designed to collect information and provide the trainee's supervisor with material for feedback, identification of his or her learning needs and possible recommendations for change.

Progression across the 12 professional competence areas is described in terms of *insufficient evidence, needs further development, competent* and *excellent*. The *competent* level reflects the standard for independent practice. While it is likely that most trainees in their first two years of training will have develop mental needs within some of those areas, they may achieve excellence in others. By the end of training, the level of *competent* is expected across all of the 12 areas.

Trainees and their trainers may use a variety of assessment tools including four mandatory ones. Two of these are externally moderated mandatory assessment tools. These are the:

- WEB-BASED MULTI-SOURCE FEEDBACK (MSF) ▷ this is designed to collect and evaluate feedback on the trainee from peers and colleagues
- PATIENT SATISFACTION QUESTIONNAIRE (PSQ) ▷ this is designed to collect and evaluate feedback on the trainee from patients.

The following two specifically designed mandatory assessment tools are designed for use in the practice and provide further core information:

- CASE-BASED DISCUSSION (CBD) ▷ this is a structured interview designed to assess the trainee's clinical and professional judgement in cases selected for discussion by the trainee
- CONSULTATION OBSERVATION TOOL (COT) ▷ this is a tool designed to help trainers to assess a consultation, and is based on summative assessment and previous

MRCGP video criteria. This observation can be done in real time with the assessor sitting in on the consultation or by videotape analysis of a consultation. Note that in secondary care placements a *mini-CEX* assessment tool will be used for this.

Other, optional, assessment tools have been designed for the trainee and trainer to use to gather further evidence of performance. These include practice audit, significant event analysis and referrals and prescribing analysis. There will also be evidence recorded through direct observation of the trainee by the trainer using a Clinical Supervisor's Report (CSR) when in secondary care.

The annual review

Trainees are required to have an annual review each year of their three-year training programme. This is a summative evaluation based on the evidence collected for WPBA. The process involves feedback to the trainee and from the trainee to the trainer. It ensures that the training and experience lead appropriately to the next phase of training. It involves setting goals and objectives, and planning the next phase of training or, if at the end of training, planning for continuous professional development (CPD).

Collecting evidence

Prior to each review, the trainee is required to collect a number of pieces of evidence to support judgements that will be made about their progress. The minimum data set required is shown in Table 2.1.

TABLE 2.1 **Minimum data set**	
Specialty Training Year 1	**Specialty Training Year 3 (primary care)**
Minimums prior to six-month review: ■ 3 × COT or mini-CEX ■ 3 × CbD ■ 1 × MSF, five clinicians only ■ DOPS, if in secondary care ■ Clinical Supervisor's Reports, if in secondary care	Minimums prior to 30-month review: ■ 6 × CbD ■ 6 × COT ■ 1 × MSF
Minimums prior to 12-month review: ■ 3 × COT or mini-CEX ■ 3 × CbD ■ 1 × MSF, five clinicians only ■ 1 × PSQ, if in primary care ■ DOPS, if in secondary care ■ Clinical Supervisor's Reports, if in secondary care	Minimums prior to 34-month review: ■ 6 × CbD ■ 6 × COT ■ 1 × MSF ■ 1 × PSQ
Specialty Training Year 2	**Or Specialty Training Year 3** **(half primary and half secondary)**
Minimums prior to 18-month review: ■ 3 × COT or mini-CEX ■ 3 × CbD ■ PSQ, if not completed in ST1 ■ DOPS, if in secondary care ■ Clinical Supervisor's Reports, if in secondary care	Minimums prior to 30-month review: ■ 6 × CbD ■ 3 × COT ■ 3 × mini-CEX ■ 1 × MSF
Minimums prior to 24-month review: ■ 3 × COT ■ 3 × CbD ■ PSQ, if not completed in ST1	Minimums prior to 34-month review: ■ 6 × CbD ■ 3 × COT ■ 3 × mini-CEX ■ 1 × MSF ■ 1 × PSQ

In this chapter we have outlined the development of the new GP curriculum and the assessment process. Subsequent chapters will look at each of the components within the assessment process in more depth.

REFERENCES

1. WONCA Europe. *The European Definition of General Practice/Family Medicine* London: WONCA Europe, 2005.

2. General Medical Council. *Good Medical Practice* (third edn) London: GMC, 2001.

3. Campbell L M, Murray T S. Summative assessment of vocational trainees: results of a 3-year study *British Journal of General Practice* 1996; **46**: 441–4.

4. Information on the Applied Knowledge Test, www.rcgp.org.uk/the_gp_journey/nmrcgp/akt.aspx [accessed December 2007].

5. Information on the Clinical Skills Assessment, www.rcgp.org.uk/the_gp_journey/nmrcgp/csa.aspx [accessed December 2007].

6. Information on the Workplace-Based Assessment, www.rcgp.org.uk/the_gp_journey/nmrcgp/wpba_and_eportfolio.aspx [accessed December 2007].

3 Reconnecting learning and assessment

The content and function of the e-portfolio

Nav Chana

Contemporary educational thinking has shown the importance of the learner making an active contribution to the learning process.[1] Involving trainees in their assessments is also acknowledged as an important principle,[2] but achieving this has often been more difficult in designing assessment programmes.

As we will see in Chapter 7, it is imperative that assessment focuses on evaluating important attributes rather than what seems easiest to assess.[3] Arguably, hitherto, learning and assessment in medicine have been separate activities often promoting superficial learning.

In designing a new assessment system, the principle that assessment should be an integral part of the curriculum has been paramount. Trainees (and trainers) should know exactly what is expected of them, and have the opportunity to demonstrate attainment over time and in a variety of contexts.[4]

Any assessment process is more valid the closer that we get to what we wish to assess. Authenticity is particularly important when it comes to assessing doctors because medical expertise appears to be domain specific and contextual.[5] Doctors simply do not behave in a stable and consistent way across clinical cases where different contextual issues come into play.[6] Therefore observing doctors in real-life situations becomes more important, allowing the collation of multiple snapshots of performance to give a global and holistic perspective of the learner.

So, what's all this got to do with the e-portfolio? The answer is simple: the e-portfolio is the portal by which 'a dossier of evidence is collected over time, that demonstrates a doctor's education and practice achievements'.[7]

The e-portfolio acts to prompt, record and summarise assessment of GPStRs throughout their training programme, including their hospital posts. Trainers and clinical supervisors in hospital settings will need to become familiar with the e-portfolio. Those consultants who have worked with trainees in the Foundation Programme will find the tool very familiar, because the RCGP e-portfolio was developed by the same team that developed the one for the Foundation Programme.

In this chapter we shall describe the key principles underpinning the development of the e-portfolio and focus on how the e-portfolio connects learning and assessment.

Key functions of the RCGP e-portfolio

In essence, the e-portfolio describes the journey of a trainee towards the goal of independent practice, ultimately marked by the award of a Certificate of Completion of Training (CCT). Furthermore, the e-portfolio has the potential to connect with lifelong learning and development beyond training. To support learning, the e-portfolio offers links to a number of e-learning resources, useful websites, RCGP publications, etc. Box 3.1 lists the main functions of the RCGP e-portfolio.

BOX 3.1 Key functions of the RCGP e-portfolio

1 ☐ It aims to serve as the reflective learning log of the trainee, available to be shared with his or her educational supervisor.

2 ☐ It will demonstrate the trainee's progress towards covering the breadth and depth of the RCGP curriculum.

3 ☐ It will act as a repository for assessments carried out as part of the Workplace-Based Assessment (WPBA) framework as well as recording achievement in the Applied Knowledge Test (AKT) and the Clinical Skills Assessment (CSA).

4 ☐ It will act as a framework for the learning agreements between learners and teachers.

5 ☐ It will act as a means of communication between trainees, deaneries and the RCGP.

We now have a new RCGP curriculum that is the route map of learning for general practice. However, knowing what to learn is not enough. Learning how to learn and reflecting upon one's practice is crucial to establish lifelong learning.[1] The e-portfolio offers multiple opportunities for learning and reflection. We know that the place of portfolios as a learning tool to encourage reflection is clear, and for this purpose they have high face validity.[8]

Private space

The portfolio offers trainees a private reflective space to record learning needs and important learning events, make notes, etc. The Personal Development Plan (PDP) section will be familiar to most involved in education and is framed around educationally 'SMART' objectives. A screenshot of the PDP from a test version of the e-portfolio is shown in Figure 3.1

FIGURE 3.1 **Example of the PDP section of the e-portfolio**

Personal Development Plan

Viewing active only [view all] ◀ ·································

Create New Entry ✎

Date	Learning objectives	Action plan	Time scale	How will I know when objective is achieved?	Achieved	
05/07/2007 12:13:13	test	test	test	test	X	✎
19/07/2007	need to read about x (From Log entry)	get a book (From Log entry)			X	✎
25/07/2007 14:42:21	Learn about causes of chest pain	Search internet. Cuttings from journals. Talk to my GP Trainer	10 days	GP Trainer to test me	X	✎
					Create New	✎

The main sections within the e-portfolio

For the rest of this chapter we will explore the content and function of the e-portfolio, which has been designed to record information in the following sections:

- covering the RCGP curriculum
- logging of technical skills
- attainment of the professional competences within WPBA
- other functions required for certification.

Demonstrating (curriculum) coverage

The e-portfolio also facilitates coverage of the RCGP curriculum by allowing the GPStR to note 'knowledge-rich' learning episodes and filing them under the relevant curriculum statement headings. We believe that this is an important element of the design, as it provides trainees with a means of assessing how they are progressing along their learning journey. This section of the portfolio is not formally assessed as part of WPBA; ultimately, acquisition and application of knowledge will be formally assessed in the AKT. However, demonstrating curriculum coverage in this way will signpost the direction of travel, and allow feedback to be given as to areas of the curriculum that still need to be addressed.

Reviewing coverage of the curriculum as a result of log entries posted by the trainee will be one of the key outcomes addressed at the interim performance review conducted by the educational supervisor. We expect, as training progresses, that the trainee will choose to *share* certain items of contributory evidence which demonstrate that learning has taken place in an area identified by a curriculum statement. This shared log entry section of learning remains totally under the trainee's control, because he or she chooses what to share with the educational supervisor.

We anticipate that *some* entries will demonstrate progress not only within the curriculum statement against which they have been tagged, but may also be assigned by the educational supervisor against one or more of the 12 professional competences, a process we have called validation. Entries such as this therefore become items of 'naturally occurring evidence'. In other words, a single shared log entry demonstrating learning by the trainee may, with permission, also contribute as natural evidence for WPBA. Box 3.2 gives an illustration of naturally occurring evidence.

BOX 3.2 **Example of naturally occurring evidence**

The trainee prepares and presents a PowerPoint presentation on the management of acute stroke at a clinical team meeting at a practice educational event. The trainee has uploaded the presentation and filed it under the curriculum heading 'care of acutely ill people'. The educational supervisor at an interim review, with the trainee's permission, tags this as natural evidence in the areas of 'community orientation', 'working with colleagues and in teams' and 'maintaining performance, teaching and learning'.

Technical skills

The e-portfolio defines technical skills as those required to undertake physical examinations and practical procedures relevant for general practice.

This inevitably calls into question whether basic physical examination skills should be assessed given that these should have been assessed and 'signed off' when a trainee completes the Foundation Programme. The argument for unnecessary duplication of assessment effort and not increasing the assessment burden are important considerations. On the other hand, however, there is a need to check that the skills have been retained and used appropriately within the context of general practice specialty training.

As a consequence these skills will be assessed *opportunistically* within the e-portfolio, using assessment tools such as the mini-clinical evaluation exercise (mini-CEX) in secondary care settings and the consultation observation tool (COT) within primary care. Furthermore, the CSA can also assess basic physical examination skills where these are built into the assessment schedules of specific clinical cases.

There is, however, a set of complex technical skills that are mandatory for the trainee to log within the skills log section of the e-portfolio. These are shown in Box 3.3.

BOX 3.3 **List of mandatory technical skills**

- Application of simple dressings.
- Breast examination.
- Cervical cytology.
- Female genital examination.
- Male genital examination.
- Prostate examination.
- Rectal examination.
- Testing for blood glucose.

These procedures will be assessed using the direct observation of procedural skills (DOPS) tool, and the trainee will need to achieve the standard of 'meeting expectation' for each skill within the skills log section of the e-portfolio.

In addition there is a set of optional technical skills, the performance of which some trainees may wish to have assessed using the DOPS and record within the skills log. These are shown in Box 3.4 and an example is given in Box 3.5.

BOX 3.4 **List of optional technical skills**

- Aspiration of effusion.
- Cauterisation
- Cryotherapy.
- Curettage/shave excision.
- Excision of skin lesions.
- Incision and drainage of abscesses.
- Joint and peri-articular injections.
- Hormone replacement implants of all types/any types.
- Proctoscopy.
- Suturing of skin wounds.
- Taking skin surface specimens for mycology.

> BOX 3.5 **Example of an optional technical skill**
>
> A trainee wishing to be accredited as competent in undertaking minor surgery asked his clinical supervisors, a consultant dermatologist during an ITP post and his GP trainer (a GP with a Special Interest [GpwSI] in musculoskeletal medicine), to assess him in undertaking the list of optional procedures using the DOPS tool. These procedures were logged in the skills log section of the e-portfolio. His local PCT has accepted this as evidence of competence in minor surgery.

Attainment of the professional competences of WPBA

The entire framework of WPBA, which is a longitudinal assessment requiring the evaluation of a doctor's progress over time through 12 professional competences, is nested within the e-portfolio.

It is worth recapping here that WPBA will:

- allow trainees to self-assess their progress through the 12 competences
- allow feedback to be provided on areas of strength and development needs
- drive learning in appropriate areas
- identify trainees in difficulty
- determine fitness to progress onto the next stage of the trainee's career.

The derivation of the 12 competences of WPBA is covered in Chapter 8, but it is important to note once again that these have been derived from the curriculum statement *Being a General Practitioner*, thus ensuring that the assessment framework remains congruent with the curriculum.

Each competence has been defined in terms of developmental word pictures that reflect increasing expertise: insufficient evidence; needs further development; competent; and excellent. The definitions that underpin these levels are described elsewhere in this book (see Chapter 9).

It is imperative that every GPStR spends some time understanding these competences, and developing an internal framework for what the word pictures actually mean. This will require reference back to the curriculum statement, and discussion with colleagues and educational supervisor(s).

As training progresses, evidence will be collected by the trainee to attest to his or her developing expertise in each of the 12 areas. The responsibility for gathering this evidence rests with the trainee. To ensure consistency and comparability, a specified minimum amount of evidence has been defined. It is very clear that only by understanding the specification of the assessment (through achieving an understanding of the competences) will trainees be able to generate the portfolio of evidence that will enable sensible discussions about their development at the regular staging reviews.

The staging reviews have been scheduled to take place approximately every six months. At each review the trainee and educational supervisor will meet and a developmental discussion will ensue. Once again it will be the trainee's responsibility to ensure that enough information of suitable quality is available to the educational supervisor.

Evidence informing the reviews will be gathered and filed against the 12 areas using validated RCGP tools. Further information on each of these tools is provided in subsequent chapters. The tools are shown in Box 3.6.

BOX 3.6 Validated RCGP WPBA tools

- Multi-source feedback (MSF).
- Patient satisfaction questionnaire (PSQ).
- Case-based discussion (CbD).
- Consultation observation (whilst the trainee is in primary care) or the mini-CEX (secondary care).
- DOPS.

In addition for supervisors within primary care, there will also be the opportunity to record evidence not captured by a 'tool', the naturally occurring evidence referred to earlier. Such entries will need to be tagged against the 12 competences in order to validate them. In secondary care, clinical supervisors will be required to complete structured reports, which will automatically request information against the competences.

It is worth noting, once again, that the validated tools simply serve to gather information, which is discussed at the staging reviews. Although each micro-assessment using a tool requires the assessor to make judgements against certain items, the key purpose of this is to generate information that feeds into the competences and generates feedback to the trainee. There is no pass/fail for any individual tool.

At the end of each training year the educational supervisor's review will also include a global recommendation about the trainee's progress (satisfactory or otherwise). This will be made to the deanery through the e-portfolio in a process aligned to the recommendations within *A Guide to Postgraduate Specialty Training in the UK* ('The Gold Guide').[9]

Following the end-of-year review, an 'educational supervisor's structured report' will be automatically generated by the e-portfolio. This is effectively a 'summary' screen that draws from the trainee's complete portfolio and provides a summary of the trainee's placements, assessments and progress over the past year, feeding into the annual deanery panel review process.

A similar report will be generated following the final review towards completion of training.

Satisfactory completion of the WPBA framework will require attainment of the standard of 'competent' in each of the 12 competence areas. Box 3.7 summarises what happens when the e-portfolio is reviewed.

BOX 3.7 **Actions at the interim review**

At the first six-month review, the GP educational supervisor and trainee meet to review all the evidence collected in the trainee's portfolio until that point. The trainee has conducted a self-assessment first in preparation for the review. The educational supervisor has viewed items shared by the trainee and noted the assessment information gathered to date.

The review progresses through the following stages:

1 ☐ validation of log entries that the trainee has shared

2 ☐ discussion of an outstanding feedback report from the first cycle of MSF

3 ☐ review of skills log entered to date

4 ☐ judgement and discussion about the trainee's progress against each of the 12 competences of WPBA

5 ☐ agreement of a learning plan prior to the next review.

In addition, the e-portfolio also has some other functions, which we shall note briefly as these are prerequisites for certification.

Documenting out-of-hours experience

GP trainees are asked to record each of their out-of-hours (OOH) sessions in the e-portfolio. In the e-portfolio the 'OOH session' learning log entries will provide a standardised way of entering information, which will normally be tagged against the curriculum statement *Care of Acutely Ill People*.

At the end of the training programme, the educational supervisor will complete a declaration based on there being a sufficient number of appropriate OOH entries having being filed by the trainee. A declaration by the educational supervisor is then completed that will appear in the 'progress to CCT' section of the e-portfolio.[10]

Declarations

The portfolio will also require completion of a series of declarations by the trainee and educational supervisor. These will include declarations of health, probity and authenticity of information filed by the trainee.

CPR certification

The e-portfolio will contain a validated entry relating to current cardiopulmonary resuscitation (CPR) and automatic external defibrillator (AED) certification.

Completion of nMRCGP assessments

This section will include entries relating to completion of AKT, CSA and WPBA.

Providing all goes well through training, regular staging reviews and deanery quality monitoring of the e-portfolio will ensure linkage with the RCGP membership and certification database so that certification can happen smoothly.

The e-portfolio was formally launched at the end of August 2007. It can be accessed via the RCGP home page, www.rcgp.org.uk.

All deaneries have designated administrators who have issued educational supervisors, trainers and trainees with log-in details and a password to access the e-portfolio.

Help and advice are available through the e-portfolio or by e-mail to the central e-portfolio team at the RCGP. Detailed guidance for using the portfolio for deanery administrators and trainees is available from the RCGP website.

REFERENCES

1. Kaufman D, Mann K, Jennett P. *Teaching and Learning in Medical Education: how theory can inform practice* Dundee: ASME, 2000.

2. Schuwirth L, van der Vleuten C. Changing education, changing assessment, changing research *Medical Education* 2004; **38**: 805–12.

3. Van der Vleuten C. The assessment of professional competence: developments, research and practical implications *Advances in Health Science Education* 1996; **1**: 41–67.

4. Swanwick T, Chana N. Workplace assessment for licensing in general practice *British Journal of General Practice* 2005; **55**: 461–7.

5. Gonczi A. Competency based assessment in the professions in Australia *Assessment in Education* 1994; **1**(1): 27–44.

6. Van der Vleuten C, Schuwirth L. Assessing professional competence: from methods to programmes *Medical Education* 2005; **39**: 309–17.

7. Wilkinson T, Challis M, Hobma S, *et al.* The use of portfolios for assessment of the competence and performance of doctors in practice *Medical Education* 2002; **36**: 918–24.

8. Roberts C, Newble D, O'Rourke A. Portfolio-based assessments in medical education: are they valid and reliable for summative purposes? *Medical Education* 2002; **36**: 899–900.

9. Department of Health. *A Guide to Postgraduate Specialty Training in the UK: the gold guide* London: DH, 2007 [Section 7: Progressing as a specialty registrar], www.mmc.nhs.uk/download_files/Gold_Guide_290607.doc [accessed December 2007].

10. Committee of General Practice Education Directors. *Out of Hours (OOH) Training for GP Specialty Registrars* London: COGPED, 2007.

31

4 Roles and responsibilities of clinical supervisors and trainers throughout GP specialty training

Ruth Chambers

Specialty training for general practice is carried out over at least three years and involves many people with different types of expertise and roles. It can also mean that at times several important jobs are done by the same person. Educators may be a clinical supervisor, educational supervisor, trainer, mentor, coach, assessor or appraiser to several people, or hold more than one of these roles for the same trainee. There are many overlaps between all these terms but the differences in the role of each are distinct.

Sometimes there is a mistaken belief that people have the skills for a particular role by virtue of their position, not understanding the specific roles and responsibilities. Sometimes one individual is expected to be a mentor, educational supervisor, clinical supervisor, line manager and careers counsellor to the same person, and conflicts of interest can arise. It is difficult for everyone involved if someone acting as the educational supervisor or careers guide, for instance, is a line manager or has authority over the trainee and can change his or her work circumstances. The trainee doctor is unlikely to trust in his or her independence and the supervisor/careers guide may act on acquired insider knowledge on a future occasion.

Table 4.1 distinguishes some of the most commonly used roles that may be adopted in providing supervision and personal and professional development and support for trainee doctors. There is often confusion over what differentiates the terms and descriptions from each other, and you may feel that at times your roles bring ticks in other boxes in this table.

Role of clinical supervisors

Clinical supervisors oversee the day-to-day work of the GP specialty registrar (GPStR). Both trainee and clinical supervisor should at all times be aware of their responsibilities for the safety of patients in their care. They will be the GPStR's initial point of contact in issues relating to the specific post. They are expected to hold regular formative meetings with their GPStR – at least at the beginning, middle and end of their placement. Clinical supervisors will carry out or delegate Workplace-Based Assessments (WPBAs), and write an end-of-

TABLE 4.1 Differentiating your roles

Role	Characteristics of role and primary responsibilities				
	One to one	Management led	Personal development	Professional development	Makes a judgement
Mentor	✓		✓	✓	
Educational supervisor	✓			✓	✓
Assessor	✓/–	✓		✓	✓
Clinical supervisor	✓		✓	✓	✓
Appraiser	✓	✓		✓	

placement Clinical Supervisor's Report (CSR) to be recorded in the trainee's e-portfolio. Hospital clinical supervisors are required to be trained for their role and are encouraged to have ongoing joint learning with colleagues from primary care (see descriptor of role on www.rcgp.org.uk/the_gp_journey/nmrcgp/clinical_supervisors.aspx).

A clinical supervisor is an experienced person who supports the trainee doctor and who aims to develop knowledge and competence, encourage self-assessment and analytical and reflective skills, and ensure patient safety in complex clinical situations. The clinical supervisor is the clinical educator responsible for teaching and supervising the GPStR in training in the individual attachment – in hospital this is the responsible consultant and in general practice the GP trainer.

See Chapter 2 for more specific guidance on the various educational duties you will be performing as a clinical supervisor where your feedback is important – such as WPBAs and mini-clinical evaluation exercises (mini-CEXs) reviews. From this we can see that as a clinical supervisor you should be appropriately trained to teach, provide feedback and undertake competence assessment of trainees.

Role of educational supervisors

Each GPStR has a GP educational supervisor who will oversee his or her progress throughout the entire training programme. Educational supervisors will hold a structured review meeting with the GPStR every six months and will review the GPStR's learning portfolio. The educational supervisor assesses progress on the basis of workplace-based evidence collected by the GPStR. The educational supervisor will conduct the GPStR's appraisals. This generates a learning plan and can also be used to identify those GPStRs in difficulty. These regular reviews do not replace formative meetings with clinical supervisors.

These are some of a GP educational supervisor's activities:

- overseeing and monitoring the trainee's progression through training
- undertaking reviews based on the assessment evidence presented
- liaising with clinical supervisors and programme directors
- carrying out regular appraisal
- completing the annual WPBA report for the annual review of competence progression (ARCP).

An educational supervisor takes more of an overview and is the educator responsible for ensuring that the GPStR receives appropriate training and experience throughout his or her three-year specialty training programme. Ideally it will be the same person throughout the three years, although local constraints may have to be taken into account.

A *mentor* will have mutual trust and respect in a supportive yet challenging relationship with a trainee doctor. A mentor should not be put in the position of undertaking assessments or appraisals of a mentee as this may undermine his or her relationship and create a conflict of interest.

An *appraiser* (as the term is used in the NHS) conducts a professional conversation with another person and gives constructive feedback about his or her performance in relation to personal and organisational goals, on behalf of an employing organisation. Appraisers may provide assistance in progression to those goals. For the GPStR this may be a clinical or educational supervisor at any given time.

An *assessor* conducts an assessment on another individual to identify the presence or absence of quality standards. This may involve a judgemental or value-free ascertainment of the extent to which standards have been attained by the individual.

Giving feedback

We all need to get feedback from others on what we do and how we behave so that we fit well into society, family life and our workplace. Feedback on all aspects of a student's period through medical school, then his or her track through trainee years, is a critical component of his or her training. We know that medical students who are poor at self-assessment stay that way throughout the course without the right intervention,[1] and that students are likely to overestimate their skills in their clinical work with patients.[2] It seems that those most likely to overestimate their skills are the least skilled.[3] Constructive feedback can improve learning outcomes and enable students to develop a deeper approach to their learning and improve competence, at least in the short term.[4]

Effective feedback will enable the doctor to gain his or her certificate of completion of specialty training with the kinds of attributes and behaviour, knowledge and skills, to be that consistently good all-round general practitioner whom we all hope to have as our own GP. He or she will be able to tolerate uncertainty to some extent whilst practising in a safe way, minimising risks to patients' health and wellbeing, and learning from error and others' feedback.

One of the most common findings in investigations about doctors whose performance gives others cause for concern is their lack of insight as to themselves and others at work.[2] Therefore, proactive feedback throughout doctors' medical training and career should help to increase their awareness of how they practise and hopefully address and prevent any underperformance.

The first stage in developing this insight is to encourage internal self-checking by trainee doctors – through self-assessment and learning from what went well and not so well. This requires a sophisticated level of reflective practice and Chapter 16 has some further details on how this might be encouraged.

Feedback might be from:

1 ◊ an educational supervisor, clinical supervisor, tutor or interested colleague on a one-to-one basis
2 ◊ patients – individual patients, or selected groups
3 ◊ colleagues at work, both peers – the GPStRs' colleagues – as well as the multidisciplinary team where the hierarchal structures provide a different sort of feedback
4 ◊ the organisation, to the team in which the doctor works, comparing outputs and outcomes relating to service delivery with those from other similar teams or trusts, for instance, and to the GPStR personally in respect of his or her educational attainment, including awards from higher education.

That feedback might be informal and *ad hoc* on a day-to-day basis – for instance a clinical supervisor might point out weaknesses or recognise a job well done in everyday interaction with the GPStR, or a patient might make a suggestion for improvement, or thank the trainee specifically for his or her help. Also, the feedback might emanate from a structured exercise that is run for that purpose, such as multi-source feedback (MSF) exercises with colleagues, or the formal annual assessments of the trainee's performance and learning.

In this chapter we will review the principles and types of feedback. Later chapters expand on specific examples that have been incorporated in the WPBA package in more depth.

Constructive feedback to a trainee doctor on a one-to-one basis

In essence, feedback should contain specific examples of where performance needs to be improved balanced by other areas in which the trainee has done well, all the while being encouraging in tone.[5] Your feedback will help to develop your trainee to move clockwise around the competence cycle – see Figure 4.1.

FIGURE 4.1 **Development of expertise (competence cycle)**

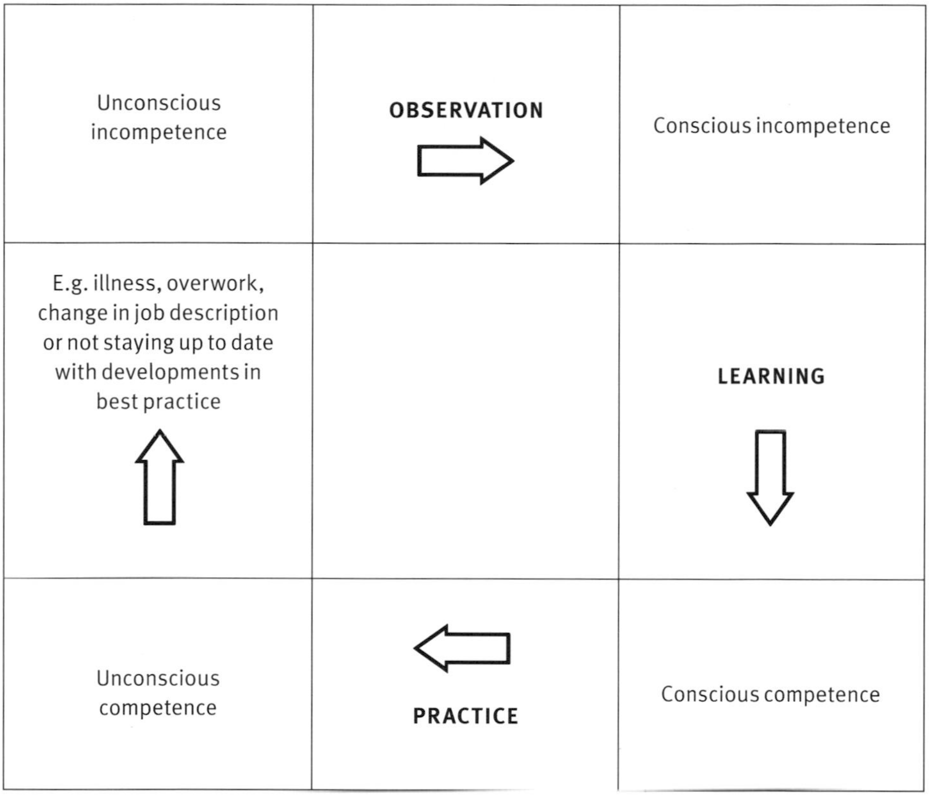

Unconscious incompetence	**OBSERVATION** ⇨	Conscious incompetence
E.g. illness, overwork, change in job description or not staying up to date with developments in best practice ⇧		**LEARNING** ⇩
Unconscious competence	⇦ **PRACTICE**	Conscious competence

Starting in the top left-hand quadrant in Figure 4.1 your trainees may be unaware of their shortcomings in a particular task until something happens to make them become consciously incompetent (top right-hand quadrant). That something might be your feedback or maybe a remark by a patient or colleague or a shortcoming they themselves realise. They are likely to feel uncomfortable about their inadequacy, so your support and encouragement will be key to helping them to learn to improve in a positive way so as to become consciously competent. They reach a stage where they know how to do something and are competent in familiar circumstances. With practice and experience they can become expert – being able to apply and modify their knowledge and skills in new situations that they may never have met before. You should continue to give feedback on performance to your trainees even though you judge them to be competent as they strive to be consistently good, and continuously reflect on their own practice.

It is possible to move back to unconscious incompetence from the position of expertise, in the direction of the bold arrow – if maybe the trainee becomes ill, or fails to keep up to date or is just too pressured by an excessive workload.

The general rules for giving constructive feedback are:

1 ◊ focusing on describing the trainee's behaviour rather than your interpretation of how you think he or she has acted
2 ◊ giving specific examples of good performance and not so good behaviour
3 ◊ being non-judgemental and impartial, rather than presenting biased views
4 ◊ referring to behaviour or aspects of performance that can be changed
5 ◊ emphasising the positives rather than the negatives; making positive suggestions in relation to negative aspects or criticism
6 ◊ checking your views against those of others to get their perspectives too.

The Pendleton model[6] is one approach to giving constructive feedback in a supportive manner, with good points first, which you could use to discuss with your trainee how he or she has done in relation to practical skills, consultations, case presentations, etc. So you would follow the sequence:

1 ◊ the trainee goes first and performs the activity
2 ◊ questions are then allowed to clarify facts
3 ◊ the trainee then describes what he or she thought was done well
4 ◊ you say what you thought was done well
5 ◊ the trainee then describes what was not done so well and could be improved
6 ◊ you say what was not done so well and suggest ways for improvement.

There are other good models for giving constructive feedback[5] but essentially all include feedback on trainees' strengths as well as their weaknesses, aiming to improve their competence and boost their motivation to learn and practise to high standards.

Of course, giving constructive feedback is not a stand alone skill. Other associated skills vital in an educational or clinical role come into play too – such as the ability to be an active listener and to motivate learners.

Feedback from patients – individual patients or selected groups

It is possible to develop teaching exercises, perhaps involving role-players, so that trainees receive structured feedback from patients. An example would be a communications skills tutorial where lay people simulate patients and are coached in giving constructive feedback to the trainee doctors taking part. That can be very powerful and the learning can be further enhanced by watching a video of the patient simulation exercise, looking back at the event after the trainee has received his or her feedback. You might repeat the exercise together later, looking at how much better the trainee performs second time round. The video might be of a series of real-life consultations that you critique and discuss using the Pendleton model of giving feedback – considering the clinical matters as well as consultation style, non-verbal behaviour, etc. It seems as if detailed criteria and video feedback to students may improve their self-assessment skills too.[7]

Suggestion boxes in a clinical setting can be the source of valuable, thought-provoking comments made by patients. Reception or ward staff can encourage patients to use suggestion boxes in a positive way, and not just for relaying complaints. Then the ward or practice manager can extract comments and suggestions relating to trainees, and feed these back as part of a constructive discussion, as noted above.

Supervisors can encourage trainees to record individual patients' comments, and collect cards of appreciation – they can help to reinforce the good aspects of their consultation skills and relationships, and may demonstrate a trend or theme that they want to develop. However, these types of comments from patients are haphazard. More robust feedback, representing the views of all patients, rather than just those moved to comment because of a particular grievance, can be gathered though the use of a patient survey. (Chapter 12 expands in further detail about this.)

Patient satisfaction surveys can give feedback on various areas of a trainee's work that a clinical or educational supervisor or trainer might not focus on. One person, such as the practice or ward manager, clerical assistant or secretary, should organise the survey. Tried and tested questionnaires should be used as they are valid and reliable, rather than designing a personal version that might have flaws or ambiguous questions. The results should form the basis of a discussion with a trainee on how to improve his or her consultation style or other areas of practice. Several patient surveys have been developed in addition to the one that has been incorporated as part of WPBA.[8] These include the following:

- the Sheffield Patient Assessment Tool (SHEFFPAT) was initially developed for use in paediatrics, but has been used more widely in hospital and general practice. It measures the quality of the consultation[8]
- the Doctors' Interpersonal Skills Questionnaire (DISQ) gives practitioners structured patient feedback on their interpersonal skills within consultations; these include listening and explanation skills, warmth of greeting and respect for the patient. Patients can add their comments on how to improve the service. Fifty consecutive patients are given the questionnaire after their consultation; results include comparisons with peers. There has been a national initiative to encourage GP registrars to participate in feedback from a DISQ survey[8]
- the General Practice Assessment Questionnaire (GPAQ) (www.gpaq.co.uk) gathers feedback about GPs and measures components of their quality of primary care. It measures communication and interpersonal skills and engagement, as well as access and organisation. It can be administered by post or handed out after a consultation[8]
- the NHS Patient Survey Programme in England is run by local NHS trusts asking patients for their views on their recent experiences of the health service.

Results of local surveys can be compared across the country and over time (see www.nhssurveys.org).[8,9]

The final choice for WPBA was the Consultation and Relational Empathy (CARE) questionnaire. This measures the patient's perception of the doctor's level of empathy and communication within the general practice consultation. It was developed by Dr Stewart Mercer and colleagues as part of a Health Service Research Fellowship in 2003.[10]

The patient satisfaction questionnaire (PSQ) for workplace assessment in the nMRCGP was devised to be used on 40 patients on one occasion. It should be carried out in each of ST1 and ST2 years, preferably when the GPStR is in a GP post, and once again in the ST3 year. The trainee GP may choose to undertake one or more other patient-based surveys too.

The most important part of such a patient survey is acting on the findings, so you should help your trainees to interpret and consider how feedback from the survey applies to them as individual clinicians, and what changes they will make. These further learning needs and learning plan should be incorporated into their Personal Development Plan.

Feedback from colleagues

Feedback from peers is valuable – but it needs to adhere to similar principles as for the constructive feedback described above, being impartial and descriptive rather than judgemental or biased. An occasional negative remark made without thought can be destructive.

Be careful too that peers do not collude in ignoring each other's defects. Stick to the SMART mnemonic with feedback that is:

- **S**pecific
- **M**easurable
- **A**ttainable
- **R**elevant
- **T**ime-sensitive.[5]

Direct observation is a common method of obtaining feedback from peers or other colleagues – perhaps performing a task such as examining a patient, or relating to others in an aspect of teamwork. The consultation observation tool (COT) component of WPBA is one such example and this is described in Chapter 10.

Multi-source feedback (MSF), also known as 360° feedback, from colleagues is currently a common feature of a training programme. Chapter 12 gives further detail on how this has been incorporated into WPBA with more detailed information about multi-source feedback in general and the two-question MSF tool used in WPBA in particular.

MSF examines the attitudes and behaviour of an individual as perceived by those with whom he or she works – as illustrated in Figure 4.2.

FIGURE 4.2 **Participating in MSF**

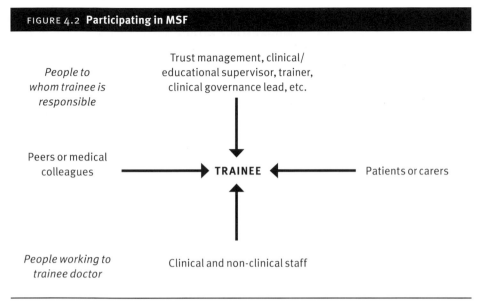

Source: Mohanna K, Wall D, Chambers R (2004).[5]

The wider the spread of people giving feedback, the more rounded the picture of their performance. Each trainee gives a feedback questionnaire to a minimum number of people in each of the groups taking part in the feedback exercise. An independent person then collates the questionnaires and discusses the results with the individual. The person giving the feedback should be trained to do so.

Organisational feedback

It can be difficult to differentiate the activity of individual doctors from that of the rest of the team – as in the Quality and Outcomes Framework or prescribing analysis in primary care. Hospital Episode Statistics (HES) attempt to attribute activity to individuals but do not reflect the complexities of multidisciplinary patient care and there may be local coding errors, particularly concerning the identities of responsible individual consultants.

Local audits initiated by trainees relating to service delivery may generate feedback about their performance versus best practice, or compare their practice with that of other members of the team, or compare the outcomes achieved by the team with those of other teams elsewhere. Although there is no formal requirement for GPStRs to participate in audit, review of practice is clearly a fundamental skill that we should encourage. By participation in audit trainees will come across further opportunities for discussion with their clinical or educational supervisor and further feedback.

There are other sources of formal feedback. Trainees may register for a postgraduate award in parallel with their GP specialty training – such as a master's degree in primary care, medical education or medical science. They may take part in certificated clinical training, study groups or learner sets. These will involve them in undertaking assignments that will be marked against the university criteria and generate feedback from others as an integrated part of the assignment and the score achieved.

All of these are opportunities for GPStRs to gain insight into their personal and professional development as they journey towards completion of training for general practice. The same opportunities also bring specific roles and responsibilities for their supervisors and require excellent feedback skills.

REFERENCES

1. Gruppen LD, White C, Fitzgerald JT, *et al*. Medical students' self-assessments and their allocations of learning time *Academic Medicine* 2000; **75**(4): 374–9.

2. Cox J, King J, Hutchinson A, *et al*. *Understanding Doctors' Performance* Oxford: Radcliffe, 2006.

3. Kruger J, Dunning D. Unskilled and unaware of it: how difficulties in recognising one's own incompetence lead to inflated self-assessments *Journal of Personality and Social Psychology* 1999; **77**: 1121–34.

4. Rolfe I, McPherson J. Formative assessment: how am I doing? *Lancet* 1995; **345**: 37–9.

5. Mohanna K, Wall D, Chambers R. *Teaching Made Easy* (second edn) Oxford: Radcliffe, 2004.

6. Pendleton D, Schofield T, Tate P, *et al*. *The Consultation: an approach to teaching and learning* Oxford: Oxford Medical Publications, 1984.

7. Martin D, Regehr G, Hodges B, *et al*. Using videotaped benchmarks to improve the self-assessment ability of family practice residents *Academic Medicine* 1998; **73**: 1201–6.

8. Chisholm A, Askham J. *What Do You Think of Your doctor?* Oxford: Picker Institute Europe, 2006.

9. Picker Institute Europe. *Making Patients' Views Count* Oxford: Picker Institute Europe, 2006.

10. Mercer S, Maxwell M, Heaney D, *et al*. The consultation and relational empathy (CARE) measure: development and preliminary validation and reliability of an empathy-based consultation process measure *Family Practice* 2004; **21**(6): 699–705.

5 Strategic and operational management of GP specialty training

Martin Wilkinson

Historically, general practice training has been organised differently from other specialties. This changed when the Postgraduate Medical Education and Training Board (PMETB) took over responsibility from the Joint Committee on Postgraduate Training for General Practice (JCPTGP) and the Specialist Training Authority of the Medical Royal Colleges (STA) in September 2005. Standards for generalist and specialist training are now the same for recruitment, training, the curriculum and assessment.

These changes have coincided with the merger of many deaneries and their Strategic Health Authorities into new NHS workforce organisations. The emphasis is on training and deployment of the correct NHS staff to meet the health needs of the local population, and encouraging new roles and skill mix.

Postgraduate medical schools for specialist training were recommended in response to the Conference of Postgraduate Medical Deans (COPMeD) and Academy of Royal Colleges discussion document.[1] It is envisaged that each postgraduate deanery will have several schools covering the full range of specialties working together to ensure standards are consistent with those of PMETB. General practice specialist training has close working relationships with most sister schools. This chapter is based on experiences of setting up the first English Postgraduate School of General Practice (PSGP), based in the West Midlands Workforce Deanery, in 2006, and discusses the roles and responsibilities within a school.

What is a postgraduate school of general practice?

This is the organisation with the overall responsibility for general practice postgraduate education within a deanery. It is responsible for the strategic planning, organisation and quality management of GP specialist training during the three-year training programme. The school's team includes all GP educators and associated administrative staff. In the West Midlands, responsible for a population of 5.3 million patients, 10 per cent of the population of England and Wales, the School is divided into five programmes, each headed by an area programme director (previously associate director) and responsible for GP training in a defined geographical sub-deanery area.

THINK □ What are the roles and responsibilities of the school? Take a few minutes to make a list on a piece of paper and then refer to the list in Box 5.1 to help you.

44

BOX 5.1 Responsibilities of the school

1 □ Workforce planning.

2 □ Recruitment to GP specialist training.

3 □ Coordination of trainee placements.

4 □ Maintenance of a regional database of trainees.

5 □ Training and calibration of educational and clinical supervisors.

6 □ Implementation of GP curriculum.

7 □ Managing the e-portfolio locally.

8 □ Quality assurance of hospital and GP placements.

9 □ Trainer approval.

10 □ Career advice.

11 □ Support for Article 11 applicants.

12 □ Support for doctors in difficulty.

13 □ Development of policies for training.

14 □ Recruitment and support of administrative staff.

15 □ Recruitment and support of GP educators.

16 □ Workplace-Based Assessments (WPBAs).

17 □ Develop strategic links within the deanery and nationally.

18 □ Research and innovation.

Previously we were organised within directorates. Superficially a school is little different from a GP directorate with the ultimate aim of producing newly trained general practitioners. So why did COPMeD recommend postgraduate schools of specialty training?

THINK □ List advantages and disadvantages of reorganising into a postgraduate school of general practice.

The aim of the school is to ensure similar educational standards across all specialties. As an example, consider the historic difference in training and approval for trainers based in hospital compared with GP trainers. Working together facilitates change by sharing best practice. A recent example of this pinching of good ideas is how other specialties have started to replicate parts of the GP recruitment process (assessment centre methodology and online application systems). What is surprising to those emerging from the relatively isolated directorate structure is that other specialties are ahead of general practice in many areas of postgraduate training. For example, the West Midlands Postgraduate School of Dentistry was one of the first in the UK to start broadcasting curriculum-based podcasts to its trainees and publish its own Wikipedia pages.[2]

Funding for specialty training has many historical peculiarities within a deanery. The differences in funding are more apparent after reorganisation into a school structure. In the West Midlands NHS Workforce Deanery the study leave budget for GP trainees in hospital has always been managed by hospital tutors, and not by GP educators. A review of this has led to all schools having the study leave budget for all of their trainees throughout the programme. All financial and administrative school structures need to be equitable.

Schools can share resources and generic training. All educators, whether based in hospital or general practice, need training, support and development as educators. A deanery can organise multidisciplinary educator training with the added benefit of cross-fertilisation of educational best practice – see Box 5.2 for examples of working together. The quotes in Box 5.2 are examples from co-workers in other specialty training schools in the West Midlands Deanery.

BOX 5.2 **Examples of working with other schools**

'Each school has project leads, for example careers, foundation training, web pages, and quality assurance. Schools can then work together to form pan-school committees in these areas sharing expertise and best practice. This ensures all schools work towards the PMETB training standards.'

'We have developed a number of posts for our GP trainees in public health, and likewise we have a number of GP placements for trainees from the School of Public Health.'

'All trainers whether hospital based or general practice based are required to attend a "training the trainers" course. The generic course is then supplemented by a school-specific "nuts and bolts" in the assessments specific to the school.'

'We are working with other schools to improve the deanery website and use this as the first port of call for questions about training within the deanery.'

'We have developed an online training package for equity and diversity training for all those involved in recruitment and selection of specialty trainees across the deanery.'

The main risk of reorganisation is the negative feeling engendered by poor change management. Sharing a vision and allowing all key players ownership is the key to success. In a large school organisation it is helpful to agree a strategic direction but allow local implementers to come up with their own solutions to put this into practice. This encourages a learning organisation where best practice and good ideas are shared.

Another challenge faced by those caught up in this time of change is the feeling of loss of autonomy or no longer being 'left to get on with it'. As a directorate we were more in charge of our own destiny, and lived in a world of ring-fenced budgets. Unfortunately the world has moved on and we cannot afford to ignore the PMETB or the Strategic Health Authority. The advantages for all specialties of having close postgraduate training links far outweigh the blinkered approach of the past.

46

The school prospectus

The starting point for any school is the policy document or prospectus. The prospectus is the result of many rounds of negotiation with the local RCGP Faculty Board, educators, trainees, Local Medical Committee (LMC), practice managers and lay representatives. This important document sets out the aims and objectives of the school and describes the organisational structure. It is outlined in Box 5.3.

BOX 5.3 Important topics covered in the school of general practice prospectus

- Basic specialist training for general practice – a three-year structure.
- What is a postgraduate school of general practice?
- Responsibilities of a postgraduate school of general practice.
- The executive board.
- Programmes.
- Duties of the programme director.
- Administrative support.
- Quality assurance.
- Job description – head of school.
- Job description – programme director.

Setting up a postgraduate school is an opportunity to revise, update and collate all past policies relating to general practice education that are tucked away in filing cabinets, folders and computer hard drives, including national and locally generated processes, and put them on the school website. At this point the school can also contact heads of other schools and scan their websites for useful documentation that could be updated with the appropriate acknowledgement. There is no point reinventing the wheel!

Management of the postgraduate school of general practice education

Our school has an *executive board* that is the strategic and operational unit of the Postgraduate School of General Practice. There is representation on the board from each of the programmes within the school. The Director of Postgraduate GP Education is the Chair of the Executive Board, and may be also the head of the school unless this is delegated to the Deputy Director. The executive board also has representatives from the RCGP, LMC, lay people and universities. The head of the school along with all other specialty heads reports to the deanery board of medical and dental training, chaired by the dean.

47

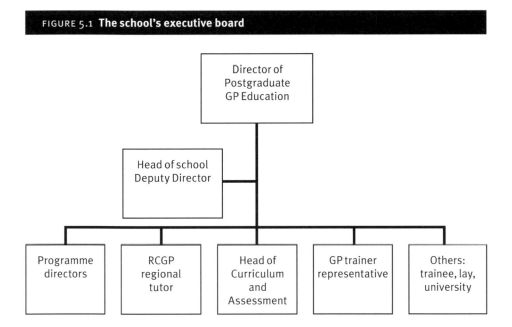

FIGURE 5.1 **The school's executive board**

A programme is a subset of the school within the deanery. Programmes are organised geographically and developed to be sensitive to local needs. Each programme has GPStRs or trainees in years ST1, ST2 and ST3, and all the programmes together form the school. A programme can choose to support the GP curriculum in their own way in response to local health needs, resources and expertise.

Induction is a programme responsibility, and it is important that trainees should receive induction to the school, trust and clinical specialty, whether based in general practice or in a hospital. The first-year induction is particularly important when the feeling of belonging to a programme of training specifically geared towards general practice will be developed. The size of the programme determines the number of GP training posts that need to be provided. So a school of 1000 GPStRs with 333 in each year could be split into five programmes of 200 trainees with 67 per year.

THINK ☐ If the school size is 1000, and there are five equal programmes, how many general practice placements do you require in each programme if all trainees spend 18 months in general practice?*

Each programme has an associate dean (or director) who manages the activity of the GP educators or programme directors within the programme. The associate dean appoints and supports the development of programme directors, GP trainers and clinical supervisors within the programme.

The main responsibility for supporting teaching and learning is with the programme directors and trainers. Educational supervision of trainees is provided by a GP trainer during the full three years of the programme. Clinical supervision in hospital posts remains the responsibility of the supervising consultant and in general practice the GP trainer. Training and calibration of educational and clinical supervisors is a school responsibility supported by a senior representative of the RCGP. In the West Midlands we have called this post the RCGP regional tutor, but the RCGP is developing a national group of senior RCGP advisers or assessors. Trainers continue to gain professional support in trainers' workshops and have representation on the executive board of the school.

THINK ☐ List the responsibilities of a programme director in your deanery and compare with the list below.

BOX 5.4 **Suggested roles for programme directors**

- Educational intervention and support.
- Induction of trainees.
- Courses based on the GP curriculum.
- Facilitation of learning sets.
- Trainers' workshops.
- Support and calibration of clinical and educational supervisors.
- Recruitment of GP specialty trainees.
- Assessment panels.
- Career advice.
- Foundation training.
- Primary Care Trust (PCT) liaison.
- Multidisciplinary training.
- Quality assurance.
- Management of training placements within the programme.
- Flexible training.

---

* Answer: 100 per programme (half the time spent in general practice).

48

Annual review of competence progression

Structured postgraduate medical training is dependent on having a clearly laid out curriculum that includes the standards and competences to practice, an assessment strategy to know whether those standards have been achieved and an infrastructure that supports a training environment within the context of service delivery.[3]

49

The three elements of appraisal, assessment and annual planning form the basis of the annual review of competence progression (ARCP) within the school (see Figure 5.2) and the process of decision making is formalised by convening deanery outcome panels within each programme.

FIGURE 5.2 **The three key elements of support for trainees**

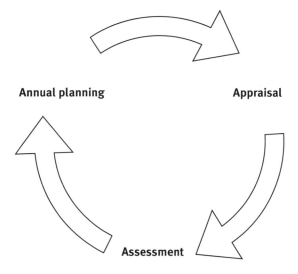

Annual planning   Appraisal

Assessment

In the West Midlands, there is one deanery assessment panel per programme. Membership of each deanery assessment panel includes the area programme director, plus representatives from local primary care medical educators, the RCGP and the head of school. The panels meet annually to review the progress of every trainee in the school. For most GPStRs, this will not be a face-to-face meeting but a review of the e-portfolio evidence. The panel makes a more in-depth assessment of those trainees who have problems identified by their educational supervisor. Most of these latter are managed within the programme by agreeing suitable short-term educational objectives or additional support.

Decisions about repeating training or intercalated remedial training will require the head of school to be part of the panel. A face-to-face meeting for these trainees takes place after the panel has made a decision. For quality assurance 10 per cent of e-portfolios are sampled by a layperson appointed by the deanery with a GP educator from another programme (or deanery).

There are a number of possible outcomes of the deanery assessment panel's ARCP for each GPStR (see Figure 5.3). As with any decision-making body within the deanery the trainee has a right of appeal to the dean, and a formal written appeals policy is agreed for all schools of postgraduate training.

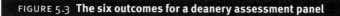

FIGURE 5.3 **The six outcomes for a deanery assessment panel**

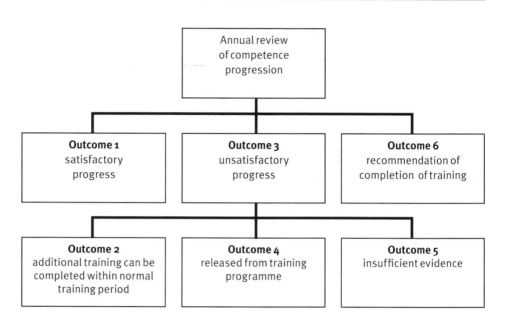

A summary of progression through GP specialty training is shown in Figure 5.4, taken from the RCGP website.

Quality assurance and quality management

There are two elements to quality control of the school training programme – *quality assurance* and *quality management*. These are summarised in Box 5.5. Quality management is the responsibility of the deanery to ensure the specialty training meets PMETB standards. The PMETB quality assures training by undertaking a number of activities to establish confidence in the training provided by a deanery.

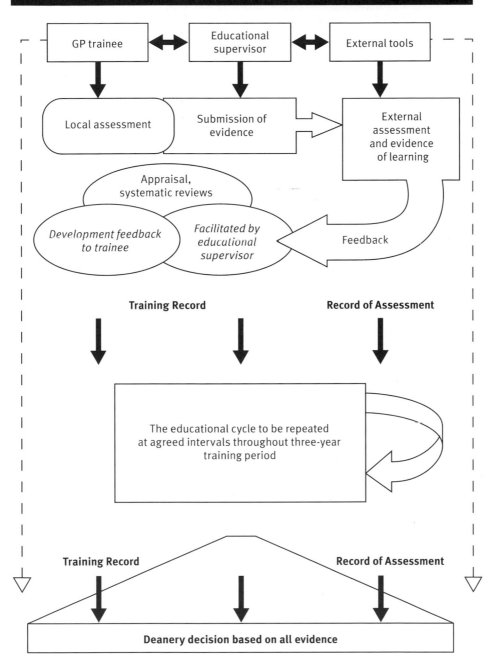

FIGURE 5.4 **Progression through GP specialty training**

> **BOX 5.5 Quality assurance and quality management**
>
> *Quality assurance (QA)* is the activity undertaken by the PMETB to provide the evidence needed to establish confidence among all concerned, that specialty training in all deaneries is being performed effectively. This includes:
>
> - targeted and focused visits to the postgraduate deaneries
> - approval process of training programmes, posts and trainers
> - national surveys of trainers and trainees
> - approval of the GP curriculum and nMRCGP.
>
> *Quality management (QM)* is the process undertaken by a deanery to ensure that all providers of specialty training conform to the PMETB standards based on data collected and outcomes. This includes:
>
> - job evaluation surveys
> - significant events
> - training practice visits
> - annual review of assessment panels.

The PMETB has introduced 'light touch' processes that rely on sampling and targeted visiting. The same methodology is also being introduced by deaneries to reduce the burden of too many quality assurance visits (often referred to as 'polyvisitosis') by deaneries and other NHS bodies.

The PMETB National Trainee Survey[4] was introduced in 2005 and first published in 2006. The aim of the survey is to measure to what extent PMETB generic standards for training are being met and to support quality assurance of postgraduate training in the UK. The national data set will be used to monitor the quality of training from providers over time. All trainees in the UK are surveyed annually by a questionnaire asking their opinion of their training. This snapshot provides information from all GPStR including general practice but excluding foundation training. The information is provided in a number of formats that allow further analysis at a deanery level and comparisons can be made between deaneries, schools, programmes, hospital trusts and Primary Care Trusts. At a deanery level the National Trainee Survey is used to develop action plans and target visiting of hospital and general practice placements.

To supplement the annual PMETB snapshot, most deaneries have regular job evaluation surveys to gather trainees' feedback after every post. The job evaluation surveys are also based on PMETB generic standards for training but can include any local standards. The post-evaluation forms are submitted by post or electronically. This provides an ongoing monitoring of posts allowing problems to be identified at an early stage. This contrasts with information gathered from the PMETB National Trainee Survey, which can be up to 12 months' out of date before being fed back to the host deanery.

Trainer approval continues to be a requirement of the PMETB. The PMETB is notified of all new trainer approvals and grants lifelong approval for the purposes of specialist training. The PMETB devolves the responsibility of trainer approval and reapproval to deaneries. There still remains the need to quality assure GP trainers and reapprove them intermittently. In keeping with the PMETB approach to target visiting, many deaneries are introducing a light-touch approach to trainer approval. This is because with the introduction of the Quality and Outcomes Framework (QOF) and PCT practice visiting there is a risk of duplication of practice visiting. An example of one such pilot is described in Box 5.6.

BOX 5.6 Light-touch trainer approval and reapproval

West Midlands NHS Workforce Deanery – light-touch trainer approval[5]
The development of the new Postgraduate School for General Practice (PSGP) is an opportunity to review existing procedures. In this light, the process for approving and reapproving training practices is being revised. There is a move to a light-touch, high-trust system with safety nets in place to ensure a safe and effective learning environment. As far as possible we aim to use recording and data collection systems that already exist for other purposes such as the QOF of the new GMS contract and NHS appraisal. Recent developments in undergraduate and postgraduate medical education mean that practice-based learning has changed, and we want to encourage a collective approach to teaching and learning, where different kinds of learners (undergraduates, junior doctors, nurses and practice staff) learn alongside each other and also share in the teaching. This also translates into a multidisciplinary quality assurance or trainer approval processes.

Initial light-touch approval follows a process of self-assessment and a practice visit where all key personnel including current learners are interviewed and supporting evidence is available for inspection. Thereafter, reapproval is based on:

1 ☐ self-assessment against the published competences of a GP trainer
2 ☐ learner evaluation
3 ☐ completion of online data collection forms (including QOF score).

Training practices include education and training status in their annual practice development plan and trainers reflect on their training performance within their annual appraisal. The school provides job evaluation information from all trainees placed with the practice and comparisons with other practices. All practices are reviewed by an examination of the portfolio of evidence every three years. Practice visits are limited to a random sample of practices as well as those that give recurrent cause for concern as highlighted by learner evaluations, or the portfolio. A QOF score of less than 750 triggers an automatic full visit, or less than 900 with other concerns.

Appraisal of trainers, the so-called educational conversation between trainer and area programme director, will continue for all trainers.

Trainee handover

During the three-year training programme a trainee experiences between five and eight hospital or GP placements. It is important that learning objectives or problems identified in any post are addressed in the current or subsequent posts. The clinical supervisor is responsible for successful handover of trainees to the next clinical supervisor. This allows a trainee to build on previous experience, and address weaker areas. From a deanery point of view we can put in remedial training at an earlier stage.

To aid handover of trainees the clinical supervisor completes the Clinical Supervisor's Report in the e-portfolio. This is accessible to the next clinical supervisor. The other key feature of a successful handover is for the clinical supervisor to identify his or her successor, making contact by email or, preferably, by phone. This is more important if there are issues to be addressed. The clinical supervisor also phones or contacts the educational supervisor if there are difficulties with the trainee.

THINK □ How can trainees and clinical supervisors facilitate a successful handover? Compare your thoughts with the examples in Box 5.7. Box 5.7 contains tips for successful handover between clinical supervisors, from current clinical supervisors on the West Midlands Deanery.

BOX 5.7 Trainee handover

Ideas for a successful handover:

'In the final two weeks hospital trainees spend one day shadowing the trainee in their next post.'

'We ensure the trainee makes contact with the next placement clinical supervisor four weeks before the end of the post.'

'All those entering a four-month GP training post within ST1 and ST2 are asked to complete a contract and performers list application at least one month before the year starts.'

'As the next clinical supervisor I make contact with the previous clinical supervisor and programme director well before the trainee arrives.'

'Because of access to the e-portfolio we will have all trainees' email addresses. Clinical supervisors can make contact and say hello in advance.'

Summary

In this chapter we have compared a school of general practice specialty training with a deanery directorate model. The advantages of working as specialty schools within a deanery are to improve standards and provide efficiencies in quality management. We have discussed the school prospectus and how this sets out the structure of the school, and the importance of including all interested parties in agreeing this plan.

We have looked at deanery outcome assessment panels and their role in the annual review of competence progression.

The PMETB quality assures deaneries and a deanery quality manages their educational providers. A deanery will work with individual schools to provide a number of quality practice tools, and we are introducing light-touch and information technology solutions to gathering data.

55

REFERENCES

1. Conference of Postgraduate Deans and Academy of Medical Royal Colleges. *Developing Local Postgraduate Schools: a discussion document* London: COPMeD and the Academy of Medical Royal Colleges, 2005.

2. www.dentistry.bham.ac.uk/ecourse/pages/page.asp?pid=258 [accessed December 2007].

3. Department of Health. *A Guide to Postgraduate Specialty Training in the UK: the gold guide* London: DH, 2007, www.mmc.nhs.uk/download_files/Gold_Guide_290607.doc [accessed December 2007].

4. Postgraduate Medical Education and Training Board. *National Survey of Trainees*, 2007, www.pmetb.org.uk/traineesurvey [accessed December 2007].

5. Hereford & Worcester General Practice Education. *Trainer Re-approval – 'Light Touch' Pilot*, 2007, www.hwgpe.org.uk/light-touch-pilot [accessed December 2007].

6 Thinking about teaching and learning

Kay Mohanna

It is, in fact, nothing short of a miracle that the modern methods of instruction have not entirely strangled the holy curiosity of inquiry.

ALBERT EINSTEIN

The whole art of teaching is only the art of awakening the natural curiosity of young minds for the purpose of satisfying it afterwards.

ANATOLE FRANCE

What do we mean when we say 'he or she is a good teacher'? As learners we have very clear ideas about what constitutes 'bad teaching' and how that can get in the way of learning. But if we were to list the features of a good teacher, that list would probably reveal more about our understanding of what learning means to us than any definitive list of essential skills specific to that role.

There is some evidence that choice of teaching style is one facet of a teacher's general view about the purposes of education.[1] We can describe two categories of teachers, formal and informal. Formal teachers see their role in terms of outcomes such as examination results, demonstration of predetermined competences and vocational training. These teachers favour a structured approach. Informal teachers stress learners' enjoyment of education and opportunities for self-expression, and tend to favour discovery learning. These two types of teaching tend to map against an understanding of learning strategy that can also be used to suggest that learners tend to be either holists ('in at the deep end') or serialists ('step by step').

A formal teacher, if asked to identify how to measure an effective teacher, might be inclined to list process attributes, such as orderliness, adherence to rules and student attentiveness, and stress the importance of knowledge base, preparation of lesson plans and handouts, and clarity in setting objectives.

An informal teacher asked the same question might tend to list student attributes such as spontaneity of students' responses, enthusiasm in learners and individuality of contribution.

As we think about being a trainer or an educational supervisor in postgraduate schools of general practice, it is clear that our learners come to us with vast amounts of knowledge, skills and attitudes from previous education and training. Their approach to learning will have been informed by how they have been taught in the past, and in particular what it takes to be successful in assessments. They will be used to success in examinations and may have developed an understanding of what they feel it takes to duplicate that success.

They may also have a wealth of experience about how to make sense of and interpret events around them. But it may be that their approach to learning is one of surface acquisition of information and not all of them come to postgraduate study with the critical thinking skills and reflective practice ability they will require for lifelong learning.

Or, to paraphrase the songwriter Paul Simon, 'When I think back on all the [rubbish] I learnt at high school it's a wonder I can think at all' ('Kodachrome').

Much of current thinking about how to effectively facilitate the learning of others starts with the premise that individuals differ in the way they process and retain information. As teachers, who similarly express differences in data interpretation, coding and recall, the knack we need to develop is to appreciate and work with these differences in our learners and ourselves.

This chapter is about how we learn, how we can effectively facilitate the learning of others, and how to minimise the risk that our assessments and other interventions might have the opposite effect of that intended.

'Learning is not only or even primarily about obtaining correct information or answers from knowledgeable others ... it is fundamentally about making meaning out of the experience we and others have in the world.'[2] This quote introduces the idea of constructivism in learning. This model, famously described by John Biggs (now Honorary Professor of Psychology at the University of Hong Kong),[3] is a way of conceptualising the journey we make as learners as we start to piece together information from our senses to create a map of the world. We take our experiences, things we read, nuggets other people tell us, mull them over and try to create some semblance of order from them. Each new piece of information is weighed up against existing knowledge and, if it appears sufficiently congruent with what we already know, or has some internal congruity, it will either be fitted in or else cast aside. So each new fragment will both influence and be influenced by previous learning.

We can compare it to the role of evidence-based medicine in defining best practice. The results of even the best designed, gold-standard, randomised controlled trial should not be blindly and automatically adopted if the results are out of step with all that has gone before. We build up best practice piecemeal.

Table 6.1 compares activities in different educational settings.

The constructivist paradigm presents us at first sight with a problem when we think about the nature of 'knowledge'. A misapplication of this model in shorthand form has led some teachers to observe that there are no 'right answers', and not unnaturally this has led to frustration in learners. This is especially so when we then proceed to test them on their knowledge of the 'right answer' in multiple-choice exams. A learner would be forgiven for thinking that the healthcare field contains a lot of absolute fact, which needs to be learnt. And to an extent that is true. But Biggs's model helps explain that how we understand these facts is open to interpretation, application and context.

TABLE 6.1 **Constructivism in practice**	
'Traditional' setting	**'Constructivist' setting**
Curriculum begins with the parts of the whole. Emphasises basic skills.	Curriculum emphasises big concepts, beginning with the whole and expanding to include the parts
Strict adherence to fixed syllabus is highly valued	Pursuit of learner questions and interests is valued
Materials are primarily textbooks and workbooks	Materials include primary sources of material and hands-on materials and activities
Learning is based on repetition	Learning is interactive, building on what the learner already knows
Teachers disseminate information to learners; learners are recipients of knowledge	Teachers have a dialogue with learners, helping learners construct their own knowledge
Teacher's role is directive, rooted in authority	Teacher's role is interactive, rooted in negotiation
Assessment is through testing, correct answers	Assessment includes that of learner's performance, observations and points of view, as well as tests. Process is as important as product
Knowledge is seen as inert	Knowledge is seen as dynamic, ever changing with our experiences
Learners work primarily alone	Learners work primarily in groups

Source: www.thirteen.org.[4] Copyright © Educational Broadcasting Corporation. Used by permission.

Types of knowledge

There is a body of medical knowledge that has developed over time. The growth of what we sometimes call received wisdom within the scientific community occurs by scholarly research and its acceptance is influenced both by the track record of researchers and the extent to which that knowledge helps us solve current challenges. This knowledge is what Michael Eraut (Professor of Education at the University of Sussex) refers to as 'coded knowledge'.[5] This can be learnt in a variety of ways, some of which will include memorisation but also manipulation through application and observation of effect. In workplace-based learning this type of knowledge will be built up by reading and study as well as involvement in clinical decision making.

Other knowledge is shared among professional groups (and society as a whole) without undergoing codification. This might be illustrated by thinking about the tacit understanding of 'the way things are done' and is sometimes known as cultural knowledge. This might be learnt through observation and reflection, particularly of role models but also by examples from best practice.

Personal knowledge or 'capability' can be defined as the combined effect of all sources of information and insight that build together and create a sum greater than the parts, enabling original and creative thoughts. This can be seen as a combination of:

- codified knowledge ready for use
- knowledge acquired through the adoption of the behaviour patterns of the surrounding culture
- knowledge constructed from experience, social interaction and reflection
- skills
- episodes, impressions and images.[5]

We each ascribe personal meaning to knowledge through discussion and debate, tempered by our feelings and experience, which develops and enhances this at individual level.

What we are looking for by embedding assessment in the workplace is a way of ensuring that our GPStRs can develop safe professional practice by extending their understanding of codified and cultural knowledge to react in unique and potentially challenging situations, which might require that knowledge to be transformed in some way. As trainers and educational supervisors our role is to create a learning environment that supports learners as they create their own map of professional knowledge.

Thus constructivism does not dismiss the active role of the teacher or the value of expert knowledge. The constructivist teacher provides opportunities such as problem solving and enquiry-based learning activities through which learners formulate and test their ideas, draw conclusions and inferences, and pool and convey their knowledge in a collaborative learning environment. As the learner is encouraged to reflect on what they have learned they achieve two goals at once: furtherance of knowledge about both work-related issues and the process of learning itself. They can become more effective learners.

But this is not an intuitive activity for some learners. They can feel frustrated and unsupported unless the process is made explicit to them. Thus the role of the clinical teacher is as much to explain the process of learning as to be an expert resource.

Development of self-directedness

Much of adult learning theory takes as its starting point the assumption that adults are self-directed. By this we mean that they have developed the capacity to organise their learning to solve problems encountered in their daily life, can initiate learning strategies and activities, and build on previous experience to understand new information. However, it is not the case that at all times, for all learners, and when thinking about all types of content to be learnt, that people all exhibit similar degrees of self-direction. Some of the frustration that learners feel in an unfamiliar learning environment comes from a mismatch between the degree to which they are able to manage their own learning and the freedoms they have been given to do so.

Gerald Grow, originally a professor of journalism, developed a model that helps us think about the stages of development of self-direction.[6]

TABLE 6.2 Self-direction stages

Student stage	Teacher type	Teaching task
1 □ Dependent	1 □ Authority, coach	Transmission of facts, e.g. basic life support
2 □ Interested	2 □ Motivator, guide	Processing and application of information, e.g. learning the skills of clinical examination
3 □ Involved	3 □ Facilitator	Development of values, e.g. of healthcare ethics and awareness of professional standards
4 □ Self-directed	4 □ Consultant, delegator	Exploration of new territory such as in workplace-based action research

Source: Mohanna, Wall and Chambers (2004).[6] Reproduced by permission of Radcliffe Publishing.

Although these stages are presented as linear and developmental, students can be at any stage, depending on past experience, subject matter and current learning environment, often in a non-linear, recursive manner.

There can be as much mismatch between a stage 1 learner faced with type 4 teaching (when they can feel anxious and lacking in guidance) as there is between a stage 4 learner with type 1 teaching (when the learner can feel frustrated and angry about perceived restrictions). It is worth asking when faced with a seemingly non-participatory, lazy or obstructive trainee whether you as a teacher may have generated or perpetuated this response by not recognising his or her stage of self-direction for this task.

A particular trap for medical teachers to be aware of is the false stage 4, dependent learner. Arising from a desire not to lose face in a critical atmosphere, some learners find themselves unable to admit their knowledge gaps, appear confident and knowledgeable unless tested, and as a result risk missing learning opportunities.

So what sort of activities can we plan to facilitate development of self-directedness? Table 6.3 categorises several activities that are associated with workplace learning.[7]

TABLE 6.3 Workplace (practice) learning

Work processes with learning as a by-product	Learning activities located within work or learning processes	Learning processes at or near the workplace
Participation in group processes	Asking questions	Being supervised
Working alongside others	Listening	Being coached
Consultation	Observing	Being mentored
Tackling challenging tasks and roles	Getting information	Shadowing
Problem solving	Learning from mistakes	Visiting other sites
Trying things out	Reflecting	Independent study
Working with patients	Locating resource people	Conferences
	Giving and receiving feedback	Short courses
		Working for a qualification

Eraut has divided the factors that affect workplace-based learning into two groups, learning factors and context factors, and we can represent them diagrammatically as in Figure 6.1.[7]

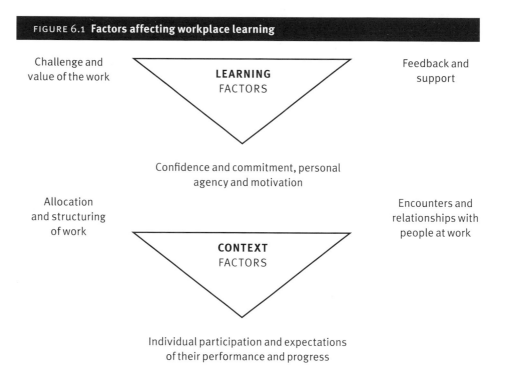

FIGURE 6.1 **Factors affecting workplace learning**

Challenge and value of the work

LEARNING FACTORS

Feedback and support

Confidence and commitment, personal agency and motivation

Allocation and structuring of work

CONTEXT FACTORS

Encounters and relationships with people at work

Individual participation and expectations of their performance and progress

Source: Eraut (2007).[7] Reproduced by permission of Professor Michael Eraut.

The principal role of a teacher can be said to be the creation and support of a learning environment where experimentation and critical thinking are encouraged, where failure is tolerated and safety maintained, and where learners are given as much freedom as they are comfortable with but as much instruction and guidance as they need.

Creating a learning culture in the workplace

Despite including plans for the ill-fated NHS University (later taken over by the NHS Institute for Innovation and Improvement) the importance of working towards developing a learning culture within the NHS – individual and organisational – was formally recognised in *Working Together, Learning Together.*[8]

In this paper a variety of development methods were described that should be supported in the workplace to enhance workplace learning – coaching on the job, mentorship, learning sets, job rotation, secondments, project work and sabbaticals, as well as formal education and training.

This acknowledged and built on the work of Peter Senge (who was Director of the Center for Organizational Learning at the Massachusetts Institute of Technology) from the 1990s:

> *[learning organizations are] organizations where people continually expand their capacity to create the results they truly desire, where new and expansive patterns of thinking are nurtured, where collective aspiration is set free, and where people are continually learning to see the whole together.*[9]

Peter Senge argued that there are five components in a successfully integrated teaching and learning culture. These are:

1 ◊ individual drivers – personal commitment to enhance individual performance
2 ◊ examination of 'mental models' – Senge suggests that the way we see the world can sometimes get in the way of learning and old assumptions need to be challenged
3 ◊ providing clear leadership about what is important and setting the pace and direction for learning
4 ◊ encouraging 'open systems thinking' so that all participants understand their role in relationship to others
5 ◊ encouraging 'team learning' so that individuals who work together also share learning opportunities to increase the chance of common 'mental maps' being developed.

Teaching style

John Biggs further helps us understand the learning and teaching process through his '3P' model of learning:[3]

- **PRESAGE** ◊ derived both from learner aspects such as motivation and existing knowledge and from teacher aspects such as teaching style and expertise, and the ethos of the learning environment
- **PROCESS** ◊ teaching and learning activities and assessments
- **PRODUCT** ◊ learning outcomes.

Thinking about this model helps us understand constructive alignment – the link between constructivism in learners (how we put together and make sense of what we learn to answer questions and enable us to perform successfully) and alignment in teaching. In a constructively aligned teaching programme, the three elements in the 3P model support each other. In particular, as we shall see in Chapter 7, being successful in an assessment implies that the learner has achieved just what was intended.

Put like that it all sounds rather obvious. However, constructive alignment rests on a view of teaching that implies a need for clarity about:

- what it means for students to 'understand'

- what kind of teaching–learning activities are required to develop those kinds of understandings
- the need for valid assessment tools to measure the competence we require rather than a proxy marker.

This is not always apparent when we look at some clinical teaching. Effective teachers should be adaptable and flexible in providing variety in their teaching activities. They will aim to match their manipulation of the teaching and learning environment to the needs of the learner and combine that with an ability to match teaching with other aspects such as the levels of expertise of the learner, whether theoretical or practical educational material is being taught and the purpose and context of learning.

This adaptability is a key skill of a flexible teacher and is demonstrated as differences in *teaching style*: the way in which teaching tasks are chosen and carried out.[1] Teachers vary in their preference for one or another style of teaching, just as learners demonstrate differences in learning styles. But just as learners can enhance their learning through application of different learning styles in different situations, even those that they are less comfortable with, so too with teachers and teaching style.

Teaching style has been defined by Kathleen Butler, educational psychologist and founder of the Learner's Dimension educational consultancy, as:

> A set of attitudes and actions that open a formal and informal world of learning to the student. It is a subtle force that influences access to learning and teaching by establishing perimeters around acceptable learning procedures, processes and products. It is the powerful force of the teacher's attitude to the student as well as the instructional activities used by the teacher and it shapes the learning teaching experience.[10]

A teaching-style self-assessment questionnaire has been developed, following a literature review on the factors that build up teaching style, which has been piloted on many healthcare teachers. This, with appropriate further reading, can offer insight into your preferred style as a teacher.[1] It is reproduced in the Appendix by kind permission of Radcliffe Publishing.

We suggest that you might complete this questionnaire and reflect on what the implications are for you as a teacher. Other advice is available elsewhere to enable you to consider further analysis of your teaching style.[1]

Supporting the new MRCGP assessment process for GPStRs will be challenging. For some trainers and educational supervisors, it will need a paradigm shift in thinking about teaching and learning. In this chapter we have looked briefly at constructivism, self-directedness, the nature of knowledge and the attributes of a healthy learning environment, including teaching style, to help that process.

REFERENCES

1. Mohanna K, Chambers R, Wall D. *Your Teaching Style: a practical guide to understanding, developing and improving* Oxford: Radcliffe Publishing, 2007.

2. Dixon N. *The Organizational Learning Cycle: how we can learn collectively* (second edn) Hampshire: Gower Publishing Ltd, 1999.

3. Biggs J. *Teaching for Quality Learning at University* (second edn) Buckingham: Open University Press and the Society for Research into Higher Education, 2003.

4. www.thirteen.org/edonline/concept2class/constructivism/index.html [accessed December 2007].

5. Eraut M. Learning in a complex world (Keynote Speech), Facilitating Enquiry Conference, University of Surrey, 25–27 June 2007.

6. Mohanna K, Wall D, Chambers R. *Teaching Made Easy* (second edn) Oxford: Radcliffe Medical Press, 2004.

7. Eraut M. Learning from other people in the workplace *Oxford Review of Education* 2007; 33(4): 403–22.

8. Department of Health. *Working Together, Learning Together: a framework for lifelong learning in the NHS* London: DH, 2001.

9. Senge P M. *The Fifth Discipline: the art and practice of the learning organization* New York: Doubleday Currency, 1990.

10. Butler K A. *Learning and Teaching Style in Theory and Practice* Connecticut: The Learner's Dimension, 1984.

65

7 Good practice in assessment

Kay Mohanna

It is very common to hear people proclaim 'assessment drives learning'. Often, those saying it are using it in a negative sense to imply that learners are more interested in 'what is in the exam' rather than learning for professional or personal development. And, certainly, in any gathering of trainers and course organisers over recent years it would not be long before the conversation turned to how time spent in completion of the video component, or the summative assessment audit, 'gets in the way' of learning to be a GP.

But it seems remarkable that we would not expect learners to worry about what is in the exam in a high-stakes professional assessment in the form of summative assessment or, now, the nMRCGP. Without success in MRCGP, learners entering training as GP specialty trainees will not leave training with a professional licence to practise.

The trick with an effective assessment process therefore must be to ensure that, by aiming for successful completion, learners are driven to master and be able to demonstrate those aspects we feel are most important. We see in the development of the nMRCGP assessment a move from 'counting the countable' to 'counting what counts' and the Workplace-Based Assessment (WPBA) component in particular is grounded in the reality of life as a practising GP. In the postgraduate schools of specialty training for general practice we want learners to demonstrate that they have achieved the competences needed for independent practice as general practitioners, so we aim to assess them doing just that. This so called 'alignment', between our desired learning outcomes and the performance required to pass, is one of the components that helps make a valid assessment.

This chapter contains some background to the principles of assessment, to help us understand the strengths and limitations of the tools in the MRCGP assessment package. The tension between formative assessments to guide learning and summative assessments of learning will be explored, the key difference between these two being the purpose to which we put the outcomes. Summative assessments act as gatekeepers to the next stage of educational development. Formative assessments offer feedback on progress. Both can act as learning opportunities themselves.

About assessments: desirable criteria

There has been an explosion of academic interest in assessment over the past few years, perhaps as a result of increased interest in the measurement of quality and standards as a policy issue in society generally, but also in education. This has resulted among other things in whole organisations concentrating on it (the International Association for Educational Assessment [IAEA] for example) and dedicated journals (*Assessment in Education*, published by Routledge three times a year). But some principles of good practice are well established.

The ideal assessment is probably not achievable in real life but we strive for certain principles to help us be as fair as possible.[1] The 'ideal' assessment should be:

- VALID ◊ it measures what it is supposed to measure, not a confounding variable and preferably not a proxy marker (if it has face validity as well, it also looks to the learner as though it is measuring what it purports to measure)
- RELIABLE ◊ it measures it with essentially the same result each time (learners with the same level of performance will be judged equally regardless of who administers it and the same performance by a learner over time will achieve the same result)
- RELEVANT AND TRANSFERABLE ◊ learners need to feel the assessment is authentic, that there is a 'real audience' beyond the assessor for whom their success is relevant, e.g., in this context, the NHS. Transfer of skills from a learning setting into practice and from one context to another is more likely to be successful when the contexts in which they are developed and used are similar
- FEASIBLE ◊ it is easy to do in terms of cost, time and skills of the assessors
- FAIR ◊ to the learners and the teachers – e.g. differences between learners that are irrelevant to the subject being assessed do not affect the result, marking is not unnecessarily burdensome or costly
- USEFUL ◊ to the learners and the teachers – e.g. it discriminates between good and poor candidates
- ACCEPTABLE ◊ in terms of, for example, cultural and gender issues
- APPROPRIATE ◊ to what has been taught and learned on the programme.

Sometimes there is a trade-off between validity and reliability; increase in one is often at the expense of the other. Consider the use of a multiple-choice paper to assess communication skills; they are very reliable since they are machine marked and equally performing learners will score equally. But such assessments are likely to have low validity. The extent to which they can measure communication skills is poor. At the other extreme we can increase validity by introducing simulated (or real) patients and an assessment by an observer. But in this case reliability will fall off since the assessment is subjective. It will be affected by assessor variability (training, experience, expertise) and we cannot be sure that learners of similar ability will score the same across all the simulated patients and when observed by different assessors.

BOX 7.1 **Principles of assessment practice**

1 □ The assessment of learning begins with educational values
To be effective any assessment process must make clear what we choose to assess. Learners gauge what we judge to be important from what we ask of them in assessments. Assessment is not an end in itself but a vehicle for educational improvement and we want assessment to drive learning in the direction of maximum effect.

2 □ Assessment is most effective when it reflects an understanding of learning as multidimensional, integrated and revealed in performance over time
Learning is the process by which we make sense of the world and ascribe meaning to our experiences. It is what our learners do with knowledge, in the performative sense, that we should be interested in. Repeated measures, looking at actual performance, over time can reveal change, growth and increasing degrees of integration of that knowledge.

3 □ Assessment works best when the programmes it seeks to improve have clear, explicitly stated purposes
What are our goals? Are we using assessment to monitor learning, to assess competence, to provide a context for learning, or to provide feedback to educational supervisors or learners? Are we looking for baseline competence, or development of excellence?

4 □ Assessment requires attention to outcomes but also and equally to the experiences that lead to those outcomes
An ideal assessment programme does more than judge the finished product. It can help us understand how individual learners learn best so we can strive to improve their whole learning experience and make our teaching more effective.

5 □ Assessment works best when it is ongoing, not episodic
This is for two reasons. First, intermittent analysis of assessment results can lead to modifications to improve reliability or validity in the way the tool itself is applied. And from the learner's perspective, effective assessments are those which monitor progress towards intended goals in a spirit of continuous improvement.

6 □ Assessment fosters wider improvement when representatives from across the educational community are involved
Assessment should be a collaborative activity between all interested parties and include self-assessment, co-workers, patients and different raters to give multiple perspectives and enhance the utility of the feedback afforded by the outcomes.

7 □ Assessment makes a difference when it begins with issues of use and illuminates questions that people really care about
Answers to two questions need to be built into the development of any new assessment tool. What do we want our assessment tools to show us and what are we going to do with the results? To be useful, effective assessment produces evidence that relevant parties will find credible, suggestive and applicable to decisions that need to be made to guide continuous improvement.

8 □ Assessment is most likely to lead to improvement when it is part of a larger set of conditions that promote change
It is not the result of an assessment that improves practice. It is change that follows from acting on the feedback coming from the assessment.

9 □ Through assessment, educators meet responsibilities to learners and to the public
We have a responsibility to the public to ensure our learners meet goals and expectations, and to our learners to ensure they continue to improve.

69

Box 7.1 lists further principles of assessment practice adapted from those developed by a group of American academics.[2]

Norm referencing and criterion referencing

Whichever assessment tool we use we need to make a judgement about what it means to 'pass'. Do we need to ensure that everyone is good enough or see how they compare with each other? Are we looking to pass everyone who reaches a set standard or are we looking to accept a certain number of passing candidates?

Norm-referenced tests rate a trainee's performance alongside others at that stage in the same cohort; judgement is by comparison with each other. They are useful for comparisons across large numbers of students or important decisions regarding trainee placement and advancement. Norm-referenced measures are designed to compare students (learner scores disperse along a bell curve, with some students performing very well, most performing around the average level, and a few performing poorly). These tests give less of an accurate representation of what each student can do, cannot give useful feedback in terms of specific strengths and weaknesses, and are not an encouragement for group learning – rather they encourage competition. An example is winning a gold medal at the Olympic Games.

Sometimes an individual mark is compared with the group average to rank students. This kind of test may be used to control entry to the next stage in terms of numbers, just as in qualifying for the Olympic Games in the first place.

Criterion referencing rates students' performance to determine whether they have achieved mastery. Very often it is done as a form of formative assessment and if we choose this we are not interested in what their rank order is so long as they have achieved the competence. Clear behavioural objectives are required to define what the student should know or be able to do and standards of acceptable performance should be set. It is most appropriate for quickly assessing what concepts and skills students have learned from a segment of instruction. Criterion-referenced assessments measure how well a student performs against an objective or criterion rather than another student. Criterion-referenced learning environments are mastery-oriented, informing all students of the expected standard and teaching them to succeed on related outcome measures. The 'bell curve' in this case is skewed heavily to the right, as all students are expected to succeed. Criterion-referenced assessments help to eliminate competition and may improve cooperation. At that same Olympic Games, an example is achieving a personal best.

Domains of learning

To be clear about what we are asking our learners to do to ensure we are setting effective assessment tools, it is also necessary to consider which domain of learning we are assessing and at which level.

In one of the earliest attempts, over 50 years ago, to produce a systematic classification of the types of learning, Benjamin Bloom led a team of education-alists at the University of Chicago to come up with 'Bloom's Taxonomy'. He divided the three areas of learning into the 'cognitive' domain (pertaining to intellectual processes), the 'psychomotor' domain (processes of physical skill) and the 'affective' domain (attitudinal and emotional processes).[3,4] More simply, this is usually thought of as knowledge, skills and attitudes.

A taxonomy is a hierarchical and orderly classification in which each stage builds on the one above. For example, each domain, proceeding from the sim-ple to the complex, can be subdivided as in Table 7.1. The cognitive domain was categorised by Bloom and proceeds from recall of knowledge to synthesis of new knowledge in original situations. The psychomotor domain was not com-peted by Bloom but work in the mid-1970s can be summarised in a hierarchy that proceeds from imitation to adaptation in unique situations. The affective domain, categorised by Bloom and co-workers in 1964, proceeds from aspects outside the learner to more internal processes.

TABLE 7.1 Learning domains and a taxonomy of learning outcomes

Level	Domain		
	Knowledge	Skills	Attitudes
Base level	1 ☐ Knowledge 2 ☐ Comprehension	1 ☐ Observation 2 ☐ Imitation	1 ☐ Receiving (listening) 2 ☐ Responding
Application	3 ☐ Application	3 ☐ Practising	3 ☐ Valuing (advocating, defending)
Problem solving	4 ☐ Analysis 5 ☐ Synthesis 6 ☐ Evaluation	4 ☐ Mastering 5 ☐ Adapting	4 ☐ Organisation 5 ☐ Characterisation by value (judging)

Attention to Bloom's Taxonomy guides our thinking about learning outcomes; the verb we use to define what we expect learners to be able to do is important because it denotes the performance we are looking for – and how to judge it.

For example, if we want learners to be able to *hypothesise*, we need to test their ability to synthesise new material and create novel solutions in new and complex, often rapidly changing, situations.

If we require them to *explain/solve/analyse*, our assessments must be pitched to allow them to demonstrate that they can integrate new knowledge and problem solve. Learning outcomes that require learners to *classify/describe* are lower-level outcomes, appropriate when we need to check they have internalised important facts and concepts, and our assessments will be based on measures of recall.

We can further clarify what it is we require of learners if we expand within the cognitive domain:

- **KNOWLEDGE** ◊ the remembering (recalling) of appropriate, previously learnt information
- **COMPREHENSION** ◊ grasping (understanding) the meaning of informational materials
- **APPLICATION** ◊ the use of previously learned information in new and concrete situations to solve problems that have single or best answers
- **ANALYSIS** ◊ the breaking down of informational materials into their component parts, examining (and trying to understand the organisational structure of) such information to develop divergent conclusions by identifying motives or causes, making inferences, and/or finding evidence to support generalisations
- **SYNTHESIS** ◊ creatively or divergently applying prior knowledge and skills to produce a new or original whole
- **EVALUATION** ◊ judging the value of material based on personal values/opinions, resulting in an end product, with a given purpose, where there may be no real right or wrong answers.

Table 7.2 helps us think about how we define our tasks to ensure we carefully construct learning outcomes to be assessed, which reflect what it is we want our learners to be able to do.

TABLE 7.2 **The link between outcomes and the words used in assessment setting**

Competence	Intended outcome	Assessment
1 □ Knowledge	Observation and recall of information Mastery of subject matter	List, define, tell, describe, identify, show, label, collect, examine, tabulate, quote, name, who, when, where, etc.
2 □ Comprehension	Understanding information, grasp meaning, translate knowledge into new context, interpret facts, compare, contrast, order, group, infer causes, predict consequences	Summarise, describe, interpret, contrast, predict, associate, distinguish, estimate, differentiate, discuss, extend
3 □ Application	Use information, use methods, concepts and theories in new situations, solve problems using required skills or knowledge	Apply, demonstrate, calculate, complete, illustrate, show, solve, examine, modify, relate, change, classify, experiment, discover
4 □ Analysis	Seeing patterns, reorganisation of parts, recognition of hidden meanings, identification of components	Analyse, separate, order, explain, connect, classify, arrange, divide, compare, select, explain, infer, interpret review, score

5 ☐ Synthesis	Use old ideas to create new ones, generalise from given facts, relate knowledge from several areas, predict, draw conclusions	Combine, integrate, modify, rearrange, substitute, plan, create, design, invent, what if?, compose, formulate, prepare, generalise, rewrite
6 ☐ Evaluation	Compare and discriminate between ideas, assess value of theories, presentations, make choices based on reasoned argument, verify value of evidence, recognise subjectivity	Assess, decide, rank, grade, test, measure, recommend, convince, select, judge, explain, discriminate, support, conclude, compare, summarise, evaluate

Formative assessment

Not everyone however agrees with the orthodoxy expressed above about outcomes.

> *Formulation of objectives to be assessed, particularly in its extreme form as 'outcomes', is naive, objectionable and patronising. It is naive because it denies the complexity of the teaching and learning task, it is objectionable because it seeks to deny the individuality of the students' understanding and it is also patronising for adult learners, because it is so teacher-centric and encourages dependency.[5]*

We have seen that assessment of learning is however paramount and the key to ensure its success is the alignment of outcomes with what it is we want learners to be able to do. As Biggs said: 'In aligned teaching the assessment reinforces learning. Assessment is the senior partner in learning and teaching. Get it wrong and the rest collapses.'[6] We can see that we need to define an approach that combines both the need for specifics in assessments and a learner-centred view of the meaning of development. If we accept that the transmission model of education does not work, then the commitment must be to teach through interaction to enable learners to construct new meaning for themselves that enables them to do the job. Formative assessment is essential in this model. It still requires us to have a clear idea of the important components of learning, but allows for feedback on specific individual understanding and performance to guide future development.

Workplace-Based Assessment (WPBA) is an attempt to do just this. It frames outcomes in terms of performance and, in the context of nMRCGP, sets performative outcomes rather than content-driven ones. With all the assessment tools, but especially perhaps with the patient satisfaction questionnaire and the multi-source feedback, the utility of the assessment rests with the quality of the feedback about performance.

In their SOLO Taxonomy (**S**tructure of **O**bserved **L**earning **O**utcomes) Biggs and Collis developed another integrative way of looking at learning.[6]

In this model, understanding unfolds from uni- to multi-structural levels. Biggs captures this advancement, which reflects different knowledge levels or forms, from procedural (understanding of sequences/skill learning) to declarative (descriptive) to conditional (knowing when to do things and why) to functioning (= a sophisticated level of know-how). It is outlined in Box 7.2.

74

> **BOX 7.2 Biggs's SOLO Taxonomy**
>
> 1 ☐ **Pre-structural level** ◊ here students are simply acquiring bits of unconnected information, which have no organisation and make no sense.
>
> 2 ☐ **Uni-structural level** ◊ simple and obvious connections are made, but their significance is not grasped.
>
> 3 ☐ **Multi-structural level** ◊ a number of connections may be made, but the meta-connections between them are missed, as is their significance for the whole.
>
> 4 ☐ **Relational level** ◊ the student is now able to appreciate the significance of the parts in relation to the whole.
>
> 5 ☐ **Extended abstract level** ◊ the student is making connections not only within the given subject area, but also beyond it, able to generalise and transfer the principles and ideas underlying the specific instance.

Assessment in this model allows us to consider not what learners say they can do, or would do, but what they actually are doing. This was described in 1990 by psychologist George Miller in the form of a pyramid.[7]

FIGURE 7.1 Miller's pyramid

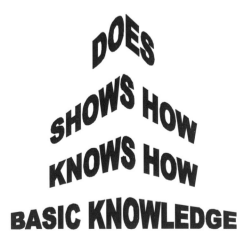

Formative assessment, feedback to learners about progress, is a two-way conversation that depends on trust between the learner and the teacher. Research shows that if learners receive an overall mark or grade, at whatever stage in the learning process, then this acts to diminish the effectiveness of the feedback.[8] Formative feedback has its greatest effect when it identifies specific areas of strength and development, and is not accompanied by any grade or mark. As soon as a mark is awarded, the effect is minimised.

WPBA in medical training scores highly in the 'good assessment stakes' by being an embedded process that looks at performative knowledge. The absence of scores and grades, although slightly modified by the need to make a judgement about satisfactory evidence, means its utility as a formative tool is high. The risk is, however, that learners, used to outcomes-based exams and summative assessment, will find the new package highly challenging and slightly threatening in the early stages. The role of the teacher must be in part to demystify the assessment package and allow the formative elements to guide learning.

REFERENCES

1. Mohanna K, Wall D, Chambers R. *Teaching Made Easy* (second edn) Oxford: Radcliffe Medical Press, 2004.

2. American Association for Higher Education (AAHE). *Principles of Good Practice for Assessing Student Learning* Washington: Exxon Education Foundation, 1997.

3. Bloom B S. *Taxonomy of Educational Objectives: 1. the cognitive domain* New York: David McKay, 1956.

4. Beard R, Hartley J. *Teaching and Learning in Higher Education* London: Paul Chapman Publishing Ltd, 1984.

5. Atherton J. www.doceo.co.uk/heterodoxy/objectives.htm [accessed December 2007].

6. Biggs J. *Teaching for Quality Learning at University* (second edn) Buckingham: Open University Press and the Society for Research into Higher Education, 2003.

7. Miller G E. The assessment of clinical skills/competence/performance *Academic Medicine* 1990; 65(Suppl): S63–7.

8. Black P, Wiliam D. Assessment and classroom learning *Assessment in Education* 1998; 5(1): 7–74.

8 Using the new curriculum to structure teaching and learning

Kay Mohanna

In previous chapters we have looked at some of the principles of assessment, what makes an effective teacher, trainer or educational supervisor, and at some of the basic principles about how learners learn. In particular we have seen that if we effectively apply the principles derived from the constructivist paradigm of education (see Chapter 6), we increase the likelihood of the following benefits:

- learners learn more, enjoy learning and are more likely to retain learning
- learners have ownership of their own learning, which enhances motivation
- learners learn different ways to think and understand
- these skills can transfer into other settings
- we can promote social and communication skills within a team setting
- we can build on learners' natural curiosity and extend this into clinical practice.[1]

We have seen that if we embed assessment into practice, we can create an authentic assessment process that gets as close as possible to the real situations in which doctors work.

The MRCGP assessment package aims for this authenticity and builds on constructivist principles. Using the Workplace-Based Assessment (WPBA) tools in particular to guide teaching and learning requires us to use everyday practice as our starting point. Both self-assessment (formative assessment elements to guide learning) and summative assessments of learning are included. Some of the new WPBA tools will act in a dual role, both making an assessment of learning and generating structured feedback for trainees on how they may improve.

Using the raw material of an observed clinical encounter (consultation observation tool) or a case described by the learner (case-based discussion), the views of co-workers (multi-source feedback) or patients (patient satisfaction questionnaire), the effective teacher will manage the learning session by guiding the learner to be able to demonstrate the intended learning outcomes. This process enables us to gather supporting information on which to ultimately base our judgement about satisfactory performance, but also guide learners to those areas we consider important for personal and professional development. This requires us to be explicit about which learning outcomes will be considered. A joint process of discussion can set these outcomes in advance – so that both the GPStR and the trainer or clinical supervisor have a say in what outcomes are to be focused on.

So, armed with the knowledge of the importance of negotiating clear and aligned learning outcomes with our learners, how does the way the GP curriculum has been written help with this? This chapter is about using the learning outcomes expanded on in each curriculum statement area to plan teaching and learning, and create a simple guide for experiential working and learning.

78

The RCGP domains of competence: six core competences for GPs

These domains of competence have been adopted from the WONCA European definition of family medicine.[2]

The first three domains have as their focal point the primary care consultation. They are:

1 ◊ primary care management
2 ◊ person-centred care
3 ◊ specific problem-solving skills.

The remaining domains are more complex and take a wider perspective, going beyond the consulting room GP–patient interaction:

4 ◊ a comprehensive approach
5 ◊ community orientation
6 ◊ a holistic approach.

All six of these are 'rooted' in an understanding of the scientific basis, attitudinal and contextual aspects – known as the three essential features.

These core competences and characteristics have been drawn from the EURACT Educational Agenda and are represented figuratively in Figure 8.1.

These six domains and the three essential features have been further subdivided to give rise to 12 competence areas, all within the context of UK general practice, to be assessed across the MRCGP assessment package.

Primary care management

1 □ CLINICAL MANAGEMENT ◊ the recognition and management of common medical conditions.

2 □ WORKING WITH COLLEAGUES AND IN TEAMS ◊ working effectively with other professionals to ensure safe patient care, including the sharing of information with colleagues.

3 □ PRIMARY CARE ADMINISTRATION AND IMT ◊ the appropriate use of primary care administration systems, effective record keeping and information technology for the benefit of patient care.

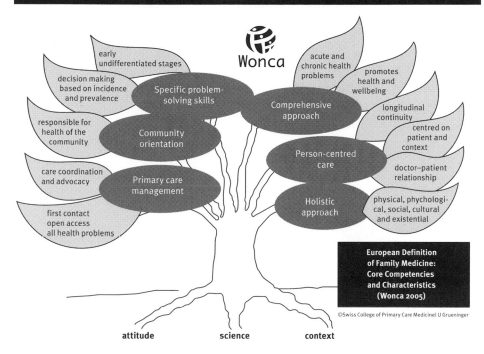

FIGURE 8.1 **WONCA Tree of Family Medicine**

Source: www.woncaeurope.org/Definition%20GP-FM.htm. Reproduced by permission of Ueli Grueninger and the Swiss College of Primary Care Medicine.

Person-centred care

4 ☐ COMMUNICATION AND CONSULTATION SKILLS ◊ communication with patients and the use of recognised consultation techniques.

Specific problem-solving skills

5 ☐ DATA GATHERING AND INTERPRETATION ◊ gathering and use of data for clinical judgement, the choice of examination and investigations, and their interpretation.

6 ☐ MAKING A DIAGNOSIS/MAKING DECISIONS ◊ a conscious, structured approach to decision making.

A comprehensive approach

7 ☐ MANAGING MEDICAL COMPLEXITY AND PROMOTING HEALTH ◊ aspects of care beyond managing straightforward problems, including the management of co-morbidity, uncertainty and risk, and the approach to health rather than just illness.

Community orientation

8 ☐ The management of the health and social care of the practice population and local community.

A holistic approach

9 ☐ The ability to operate in physical, psychological, socioeconomic and cultural dimensions, taking into account feelings as well as thoughts.

Attitude

10 ☐ MAINTAINING AN ETHICAL APPROACH TO PRACTICE ◊ practising ethically with integrity and respect for diversity.

11 ☐ FITNESS TO PRACTISE ◊ the doctor's awareness of how his or her own performance, conduct or health, or that of others, might put patients at risk and the action taken to protect patients.

Scientific

12 ☐ MAINTAINING PERFORMANCE, LEARNING AND TEACHING ◊ maintaining the performance and effective continuing professional development of oneself and others.

We can summarise these competence areas and they can be mapped against the assessment tools to give an idea of which ones can be assessed by which tool (see Table 8.1). They do however also apply equally to clinical encounters, tutorials, reading, lectures, seminars, professional conversations and more, which are all fundamental components of the learning environment.

TABLE 8.1 **Demonstrating competence**[3]				
Competence area	MSF	PSQ	COT	CbD
Communication and consultation skills	✓	✓	✓	
Practising holistically		✓	✓	✓
Data gathering and interpretation	✓		✓	✓
Making a diagnosis/making decisions	✓		✓	✓
Clinical management	✓		✓	✓
Managing medical complexity and promoting health				✓
Primary care administration and IMT				✓
Working with colleagues and in teams	✓			✓
Community orientation				✓
Maintaining performance, learning and teaching	✓			
Maintaining an ethical approach to practice	✓			✓
Fitness to practise	✓			✓

Outcomes from all these learning opportunities will be captured and gathered together in the e-portfolio (see Chapter 3). Which areas will be discussed in any individual session will of course be dictated by the nature of the information under discussion (see Chapters 9, 10, 13 and 14).

So what is the practical application of this?

Imagine it is Tuesday morning and you are about to give a tutorial. How can this structure help organise teaching and learning? Consider the scenario in Box 8.1 and answer the questions below it.

BOX 8.1 Applying the new GP curriculum

Simon Brown is 27 and requires thrice-weekly dialysis for chronic renal failure. This followed kidney damage caused by medical treatment for Crohn's disease. He has been on the waiting list for a kidney transplant for nine months. His parents are supportive and often accompany him to appointments. Simon has been cheerful and optimistic, although he recently broke off his engagement so that his fiancée could 'get on with her life'. The practice nurses look forward to seeing him on his regular visits for blood tests, which fit in between his part-time studies to be an architect. Last week he came in to see the trainee in the practice, 'just to drop off a letter to be filed in my notes'. He then left the surgery.

In the letter he explains that he has decided not to continue with the dialysis, which he finds burdensome, and 'take his chances'.

Your trainee brings this to you as a 'problem case'.

1. What might your trainee express as 'felt' educational needs?

....

2. How might you uncover whether there are any further, unexpressed or unidentified, learning needs?

....

3. Which GP curriculum competences apply?

....

4. How will you know if this has been a successful tutorial?

....

Although this is a general practice-based example, similar cases will arise out of outpatients or ward-based encounters. We can imagine that in the case of Simon Brown, in Box 8.1, the GPStR might have been working in the ward where Simon was seen and found herself in a similar situation.

A tutorial like this could become wide ranging and last an hour or more, although the amount of useful learning after an hour's discussion might be limited. Chapter 9 will go on to show how the case-based discussion tool can also be used with cases such as this. When a formal assessment is planned in this way, the assessment, complete with feedback, should last no longer than half an hour in total.

Trainers are used to managing problem case analysis. One effective formula looks something like this:

- STEP ONE ▷ comprehend the case situation (clarify facts, identify key players)

- STEP TWO ▷ define the problem (Why is this a problem for the trainee? What particular aspect is he or she finding difficult?)

- STEP THREE ▷ identify the issues (brainstorming and clarifying all the areas that are perceived as problematic)

- STEP FOUR ▷ generate alternative solutions (discussing options, alternative strategies, things we could do, discussing consequences and pros and cons of each)

- STEP FIVE ▷ make a decision

- STEP SIX ▷ take action (discuss and take advice, refer, defer, decide to take no action).

In the case of Simon Brown, our analysis might look like this:

- STEP ONE ▷ do I (the trainer or clinical supervisor) know Simon Brown? Who is his regular doctor? Do we know the other family members? What medication is he on?
- STEP TWO ▷ what is it that makes this a problem for this trainee?

Possible issues and answers include:

- the patient may be her age, or the same age as a brother or close friend
- does she wonder what legal status this letter has?
- is Simon depressed? Does the trainee know how to diagnose depression? If he is depressed, can he make such a decision to abandon treatment? Does the trainee understand that competence is decision specific?
- what level of understanding does she have about chronic renal disease and its prognosis
- what does she know about transplant surgery?
- does she appreciate the risk/likely time till onset of a medical deterioration without dialysis?
- what does she know about prognosis and treatment of Crohn's disease? And the side effects of that treatment?
- does she feel she could involve family members? Is she worried about confidentiality?
- unexpected issues may be identified by the trainee.

82

STEP THREE ◊ what issues can we as trainers identify? For example, what if the trainee has not considered a red flag such as the risk of suicide or the risk of death from acute renal failure? Other than those raised as problems by the trainee in today's situation, what other aspects can she see might complicate another similar such consultation. Can the trainer add any more?

STEP FOUR ◊ what options are open to us? What might we do next?

- File the letter and send a copy to his consultant.
- Have a multidisciplinary meeting or significant event discussion in the practice.
- Ask Simon to come in for a further, possibly joint, consultation.
- Talk to his consultant in the hospital.
- Discuss the case with a psychiatrist for advice.
- Contact our medical defence organisation for advice.
- Further options identified by you and the trainee.

A discussion of the possible foreseeable consequences of each option then follows.

STEP FIVE ◊ decide on a course of action:

1 ◊ deal with Simon's case – there is clearly a real risk of deterioration of renal function if we do not act rapidly
2 ◊ set some educational objectives, e.g. go away and look some aspects up, consider a visit to a renal unit, etc.

STEP SIX ◊ carry it out. And decide how/whether you will follow things up (clinically, educationally).

Now let us consider the same case through the filter of the new curriculum, particularly with an eye to gathering supporting information for the e-portfolio to demonstrate that competences are being achieved. The 12 competences are in italic on Table 8.2.

TABLE 8.2 Demonstrating achievement of the 12 competences

Primary care management	Clinical management	How do I find out if he is depressed?
		Are there metabolic or biochemical factors that might affect his judgement?
	Working with colleagues and in teams	How are others involved in his care and are we collectively responding to his needs appropriately?
		Should we have a significant event meeting?
	Primary care administration and IMT	Should we file this letter in his notes?
		What might be the implications if we do?

Continued over

Person-centred care	*Communication and consultation skills*	What do I need to manage this case sensitively and come to understand the patient perspective?
		Why has the patient come now?
		How do I find out his unexpressed needs and wants?
		How can I make a joint decision with the patient?
		How can I ensure continuity – for this episode, and the future, for patient and for the doctor?
	Practising holistically	What advice is likely to be acceptable to the patient?
		Is my plan respectful of his values and beliefs; and those of his family?
		Are the views or cultural values of the wider community relevant?
		What does the trainee know about transplant registers?
Specific problem-solving skills	*Data gathering and interpretation*	How serious a problem is this?
		What are the key features?
		What are the risks?
	Making a diagnosis/ making decisions	Today, at some point?
A comprehensive approach	*Managing medical complexity and promoting health*	This raises so many issues, how do I prioritise them?
		Can I delegate some of the tasks?
	Community orientation	Can I involve his family in his management?
		How are his studies going?
		Are there financial problems, and does he qualify for benefits?
		What is the financial impact on the NHS of all the possible options?
		Are there certain options he could afford?

Attitudinal aspects	Maintaining an ethical approach to practice	How do I best respect Simon's autonomy and balance this with beneficence, non-maleficence and justice?
	Fitness to practise	How do I maintain professionalism in the face of my own emotions?
Scientific approach	Maintaining performance, learning and teaching	What unmet educational needs have we discovered and how would they best be tackled?

By the end of this session, you and the learner will have identified many areas where she is performing well. You will encourage her to reflect on the discussion and she will be able to enter this into her portfolio, linked to different competences.

In addition you will have identified some areas where there is a knowledge gap. What might you do then? The strength of this system is that the assessment process identifies areas for future development within the curriculum framework, and the curriculum statement areas themselves contain a synopsis of up-to-date information for all areas, with pointers to further learning resources.[4] In this particular case it is likely that information that helps will be found in more then one curriculum statement (*Care of Children and Young People*, *Men's Health* and *Care of People with Cancer and Palliative Care*). Many aspects of general practice learning will be like that. In addition there are aspects such as dealing with uncertainty, harnessing emotions and managing complexity that are common to all and for which there are likely to be no 'written-down' answers.

The general practice curriculum statements act as a resource for learning materials for all educators as well as trainees. In relation to hospital attachments, the statements offer guidance to hospital consultants and trainees on the general practice-specific learning outcomes associated with areas of care, which are likely to differ in some respects from the requirements in specialty training. For example, a specialty trainee en route to be a consultant paediatrician needs the skill of inserting an umbilical arterial catheter, a skill unlikely to be used in the community by a GP specialty trainee. A GP specialty trainee on the other hand needs to be able to talk authoritatively to new parents about the management of minor self-limiting childhood conditions, conditions rarely seen in hospital. However, both need to be able to spot the warning signs of meningococcal disease and distinguish it in its early stages from a non-specific viral illness. A consultant paediatrician acting as a clinical supervisor for GP specialty trainees will find useful guidance in the GP curriculum statement on *Care of Children and Young People* to enable them to focus the teaching and learning opportunities he or she provides.

As the trainer or educational supervisor working with the learner who met Simon Brown, we then have one final task – to guide the learner to devise a strategy to bridge any identified learning gaps herself. If there is a knowledge-based gap, she may need to look things up ether in a textbook or online, or there may be an appropriate course. If there is a skill-based gap, e.g. problem solving or decision making, or a practical skill, she may be able to address that with more practice or discussion of cases. It might also be necessary to consider further targeted training, e.g. in a skills lab. Attitudinal aspects also have appropriate learning activities that can be mapped against gaps, for example in this case perhaps a visit to a renal dialysis unit might be arranged, or maybe a local hospice has an educational programme around supporting patients with chronic life-threatening illnesses.

Learners do not have to demonstrate that they have been assessed in all of the learning outcomes for all the curriculum areas (the GP curriculum contains over 1000 of them!). Rather, they need to demonstrate their mastery of all six core competences and the three essential features within a (representative) variety of contexts.[5]

Learners as teachers

Back in your practice, it is the following week now and having managed Simon Brown clinically and ensured patient safety, you have also considered all the learning needs that arose from your discussion of his case. You are now planning this week's tutorial. Your registrar had looked at the GP curriculum statement on *Men's Health* and has decided that there are aspects to looking after men, especially in the 16–44 year age range, that she had not realised before. She had always assumed (if she thought about it at all) that there was not that much difference in the way people of both genders and different ages consulted in general practice.

So, following on from your discussions, she has decided to put a case together for a men's health clinic. Today you are going to discuss what progress she has made. The only guidance you have given her is to use the competences of the GP curriculum to structure her planning. Box 8.2 outlines what she has come up with.

You are so impressed with her ideas that you ask her to present her work at the practice meeting, thus enabling her to demonstrate further learning in the domain of primary care management – competence in working with colleagues and in teams – and also in the scientific domain – competence in learning and teaching.

In summary, the GP curriculum, and in particular the themes or learning outcomes contained and expanded in each statement area, can guide us towards excellence by providing a structured and rigorous framework for practice-based learning.

BOX 8.2 Using the GP curriculum statement *Men's Health* to plan a men's health clinic

Things to think about when planning a men's health clinic

Primary care management
- All the nurses are female. What can we do about chaperones?

- Can the computer generate invitations to men aged 16–44 that have not been seen in the last, say, three years?

Person-centred care
- Men may be less articulate about their health compared with women – but they don't worry less.

- We know that men die younger than women, they take more risks with their health and they get more cardiovascular disease and cancer. Do they know that? Perhaps we need a poster campaign in the surgery?

Specific problem-solving skills
- Have we got some leaflets about the pros and cons of prostate-specific antigen (PSA) testing in the asymptomatic person?

A comprehensive approach
- How would the doctors feel about giving away condoms?

- We should use consultations opportunistically for health education.

Community orientation
- Do we need to offer clinics either later in the day or on Saturday mornings to fit with the hours of men who work?

A holistic approach
- The Parentcraft meetings need to move to the evenings so that expectant fathers can come.

Contextual aspects
- We have a big military barracks in our catchment area that must have expertise in men's health. Could we have a teaching session/joint meeting with the defence medical services to update us?

Attitudinal aspects
- Some men may have limited control over lifestyle choices, such as those from low socioeconomic groups, or those living with an addiction.

We can also summarise how to manage learning in Box 8.3.

BOX 8.3 **Guidelines for managing learning effectively through the GP curriculum**
1 ☐ Think of positive ways to motivate your learners. What matters to them?
2 ☐ Base the learning on learners' needs.
3 ☐ Give learners the responsibility for learning.
4 ☐ Goals should be translated into specific, curriculum-based outcomes.
5 ☐ Make the learning interesting.
6 ☐ Make learners active contributors to the learning process.
7 ☐ Give regular, constructive (high-support, high-challenge) feedback on progress.
8 ☐ Allow time, and build the skills required, for reflection.
9 ☐ Reinforce the positive not the negative aspects.
10 ☐ Remember that learning feeds on success.
11 ☐ Ensure that a supportive learning environment is provided.
12 ☐ Reward both good performance and good learning discipline.

Source: adapted from Mohanna *et al.*[6]

REFERENCES

1. Biggs J. *Teaching for Quality Learning at University* (second edn) Buckingham: Open University Press/Society for Research into Higher Education, 2003.

2. WONCA Europe. *The European Definition of General Practice/Family Medicine* London: WONCA Europe, 2005.

3. www.rcgp.org.uk/the_gp_journey/nmrcgp/wpba_and_eportfolio/collecting_evidence.aspx [accessed December 2007].

4. www.rcgp-curriculum.org.uk/rcgp_-_gp_curriculum_documents.aspx [accessed December 2007].

5. Deighan M. *The Learning and Teaching Guide* London: RCGP, 2007.

6. Mohanna K, Wall D, Chambers R. *Teaching Made Easy* (second edn) Oxford: Radcliffe Medical Press, 2004.

9 **Workplace-Based Assessment**

Case-based discussion

Patti Gardiner

What this tool is about

Talking and listening are indispensable communication skills used by hospital consultants and GP trainers when educating and assessing their GP specialty registrars (GPStR). It is no great surprise therefore that this has been incorporated as the case-based discussion tool (CbD) in Workplace-Based Assessment (WPBA), the element of nMRCGP in which such educators are intimately involved.

CbD is an assessment tool designed to gather evidence of the GPStR's capabilities across ten of the 12 WPBA competence areas that have been drawn directly from the RCGP curriculum. It does not require a pass/fail judgement and does not sit comfortably with summative/formative assessment terminology either. Rather it is one of a number of ways that GP educators will build up a rich picture of the ability of their GPStR.

CbD has great validity as it gives an opportunity to explore what the GPStR has actually done and as such sits at the top of Miller's pyramid (see Chapter 7).

It has been shown that multiple sampling is a highly effective method of assessing competence and contrasts with the psychometrically monitored examinations to which we have become accustomed where reliability is of core importance.[1] The process can be likened to a digital photograph. The more pixels we have the clearer the picture becomes. Just so with a GPStR: the more evidence we gather, even though each individual piece may not have been gathered with a robustly reliable method, the clearer and richer a picture we assemble of their competence to be a GP. It has been designed to be as reliable as possible by drawing on the experience and limited research available on oral assessment, which all concludes that structured interviewing is more reliable than unfocused random case analysis.

Rationale and evidence base

CbD was developed by a group of examiners experienced in delivering the MRCGP oral examination. It has been influenced by our extensive experience of using talking and listening in evaluation but also draws on experience and evidence from five main areas in the international literature.

Chart stimulated recall

This was described in the USA and Canada.[2] It is one of various assessment methods listed in the ACGME (Accreditation Council for Graduate Medical Education) toolbox.[3] It comprises a standardised oral assessment, based on patient cases, which measures clinical decision making, analytical thinking skills and the ability to formulate and carry out a management plan. It was found to be a highly effective way to assess clinical performance.

The MRCGP oral examination

This has become increasingly consistent over the past 12 years with the introduction of a clear structure in which the examiner prepares detailed questions in advance. Care is taken during this preparation to decide what evidence is necessary for each performance level. This has considerably improved the reliability of the test.[4,5]

Over the years the panel of examiners has identified that the MRCGP oral component explores the decision making that underpins professional judgement (see Box 9.1). This is an area that is difficult to assess in written examinations as the examiner cannot cross-examine the candidate seeking justification for his or her decisions and actions. It is encouraging that, in 1993, Elstein suggested that oral interview is more effective than written examination in 'the domain of clinical competence involved with deliberation and reflection, particularly in situations where there is no consensus about the "most nearly correct" answer, and where values and risk assessments vary considerably among both clinicians and patients'.[6] There is little doubt that oral interview is an important way to explore clinical situations of complexity and uncertainty.

BOX 9.1 **Professional judgement**

Professional judgement is the ability to make holistic, balanced and justifiable decisions in situations of complexity and uncertainty. It may include the ability to make rational decisions in the absence of complete information or evidence and to take action or even do nothing in such situations.

It requires a selection of skills: recognising uncertainty/complexity; application or use of medical knowledge; application or use of ethical and legal frameworks; and ability to prioritise options, consider implications and justify decisions.[7]

Other main areas of experience and evidence

Other experiences supporting the inclusion of CbD in WPBA are the successful use of CbD in Foundation Programme training (FT)[8,9] and by the General

Medical Council (GMC) when exploring issues of competence with established GPs.[10,11] The limited assessment literature that does exist confirms that the more structured an oral interview is, the more reliable the judgement about the candidate's competence.[12–16]

Which WPBA competences does CbD explore?

The 12 WPBA competences are summarised in Box 9.2 in the order in which they appear in the e-portfolio. Those in italics (1 and 10) are better explored using other tools and have therefore not been included in the CbD mark sheet.

BOX 9.2 **WPBA competences**

1 ☐ *Communication and consultation skills concerns communication with patients and the use of recognised consultation techniques.*

2 ☐ **Practising holistically** concerns the ability of the doctor to operate in physical, psychological, socioeconomic and cultural dimensions.

3 ☐ **Data gathering and interpretation** concerns the gathering and use of data for clinical judgement, the choice of physical examination and investigations, and their interpretation.

4 ☐ **Making a diagnosis/making decisions** concerns the conscious, structured approach to decision making.

5 ☐ **Clinical management** concerns the recognition and management of common medical conditions in primary care.

6 ☐ **Managing medical complexity and promoting health** concerns aspects of care beyond managing straightforward problems, including the management of co-morbidity, uncertainty, risk and the approach to health rather than just illness.

7 ☐ **Primary care administration and IMT** concerns the appropriate use of primary care administration systems and effective record keeping and information technology for the benefit of patient care.

8 ☐ **Working with colleagues and in teams** concerns working effectively with other professionals to ensure patient care, including the sharing of information with colleagues.

9 ☐ **Community orientation** concerns the management of the health and social care of the practice population and local community.

10 ☐ *Maintaining performance, learning and teaching concerns maintaining the performance and effective continuing professional development of oneself and others.*

11 ☐ **Maintaining an ethical approach to practice** concerns practising ethically with integrity and a respect for diversity.

12 ☐ **Fitness to practise** concerns the doctor's awareness of when his or her own performance, conduct or health, or that of others, might put patients at risk and the action taken to protect patients.

Carrying out a CbD

Preparing for the CbD

Structuring the interview improves the reliability of the judgement made. It is important therefore to prepare the discussion by identifying the competence areas to be explored, choosing appropriate questions and thinking in advance about what you might expect of trainees at the various stages of competence.

TIP

The preparation requires familiarity with the CbD paperwork, which you will find on the RCGP website[17] and in the e-portfolio. It will be helpful to have this paperwork to hand as you read the next section of this chapter.

A week before the CbD is to be conducted the GPStR will give the assessor relevant notes (e.g. a printout of a consultation, family history, drug history, appropriate correspondence or test results) of four cases for which he or she has been responsible. These should be cases that have some element of complexity or uncertainty requiring decisions. During the hospital attachment it is important that assessors remember to use such discussions to specifically explore elements of the GP curriculum. During the GP attachment the GPStR is guided to include some cases relating to children, mental health, cancer/palliative care and older adults. These might include house calls, out-of-hours experience or significant events, as well as surgery consultations. If there are particular competences that you wish to look at with the GPStR then it is totally acceptable to recommend particular material for use in a CbD. The assessor should then select two of the four cases to discuss.

STEP 1 ⟡ from the cases you have chosen and any previous experience of the GPStR identify the competence areas you wish to explore.

It is impossible to explore all ten areas in one interview as this would allow the discussion to remain superficial and would encourage it to take longer than is recommended. The attraction of the CbD is its ability to explore in depth the rationale behind the decisions and actions taken by the trainee. This is done more effectively if the discussion is focused on a small number of competences and the time is used to probe each in depth.

STEP 2 ⟡ decide which questions you might use to look at the competences you have chosen. See the 'case-based discussion notes sheet' to help with this.

STEP 3 ◊ the structured question guidance sheet offers some ideas of the sorts of questions that can be helpful when asking GPStRs to explain why they acted as they did.

MRCGP examiners found over many years that there are a number of generic exploratory questions that can be used very effectively in various areas and contexts. These are useful for looking at the various skills required in professional judgement (see Box 9.1). These have been crystallised into those on the structured question guidance sheet, but they are for guidance only. It is likely that assessors will develop other questions specific to the competence being assessed, which may be a useful starting point. The recommended structured questions may then be useful in supplementary investigation of the GPStR's justification for his or her actions.

93

STEP 4 ◊ look at the detailed descriptors of the curriculum competence areas summarised in Box 9.2. For each competence, the GPStR may be found to be at one of four levels of performance (see Box 9.3).

BOX 9.3 Developmental word pictures indicating levels of performance	
Insufficient evidence	From the available evidence, the doctor's performance cannot be placed on a higher point of this developmental scale
Needs further development	Rigid adherence to taught rules or plans. Superficial grasp of unconnected facts. Unable to apply knowledge. Little situational perception or discretionary judgement
Competent	Accesses and applies coherent and appropriate chunks of knowledge. Able to see actions in terms of longer-term goals. Demonstrates conscious and deliberate planning with increased level of efficiency. Copes with crowdedness and able to prioritise
Excellent	Intuitive and holistic grasp of situations. No longer relies on rules or maxims. Identifies underlying principles and patterns to define and solve problems. Relates recalled information to the goals of the present situation and is aware of the conditions for application of that knowledge

For the competences that you plan to look at (remember not to select too many), and with the help of the detailed descriptors, think what actual evidence from each particular case you would be expecting to find to reflect the level of performance of the GPStR. Make a note of this on your planning sheet to refer to when you are in discussion.

Important: remember that you are judging against an aspirational level of achievement – that of a competent GP, not that expected of a trainee at this stage in their training.

How to conduct the CbD

This is not an examination but is an essential part of the GPStR's ongoing assessment and so it is important that you ensure you will not be disturbed during the discussion.

Timing

During the MRCGP orals it has been recognised that restricting the time for the interview focuses the minds of the examiners, and makes them keep to the point of their prepared questions so that the candidate can be graded accurately. For this reason, it is recommended that trainers and educators allow about 20 minutes for each discussion, followed by about ten minutes to offer feedback to the trainee. This is not intended to be strictly timed but you are advised not to allow the discussion to over-run very much as it is unlikely that you will gather more evidence by extending the interview. It is more likely that extra time will be used in discussion, which may be interesting but does not help you to make a more accurate judgement of the trainee's competence.

Discussion

It can be helpful to tell the GPStR at the beginning of the discussion which competence areas you are going to look at. We would advise that the discussion is kept focused on the particular competences chosen for exploration. It can be tempting to move into a new and unprepared competence area but this may not facilitate a more reliable judgement about the GPStR as there has not been any preparation and therefore the discussion will be unstructured.

Make notes as you go and move systematically through the selected competences. At the conclusion of the interview refer again to the detailed descriptors and take a few moments to crystallise your thoughts about where on the spectrum of ability the GPStR lies. Record your assessment on the mark sheet in the e-portfolio. You are also required to make an overall judgement about how you feel the GPStR has performed generally in handling the case. This assessment will be informed by the evidence you have obtained during your discussion.

Experience of examiners: the paperwork may feel bewildering at first, particularly when trying to understand and assimilate the various word pictures, i.e. the detailed descriptors for each competence area as well as the performance-level developmental word pictures. MRCGP oral examiners also had two sets of word pictures to use. Their universal experience was that when they started examining they frequently referred to them, but very quickly found that they became so familiar with the word pictures that judgements became much quicker and easier.

Feedback

The second part of the CbD process is to offer feedback to the GPStR. This may include affirmation of good professional judgement, appropriate action and sound justification. It is, however, important to include recommendations for further training. These should then be distilled with the GPStR into agreed actions. We would once again recommend that you try to do this within the recommended ten minutes.

95

Experience of trainers: in Northamptonshire, trainers began to use the CbD in 2006. They found it a very informative tool that they quickly incorporated into their teaching and their mid-term assessments. With use they have become quite familiar with the paperwork and have much more confidence in making assessment judgements.

Some have found it so helpful that they also use it as a tool to identify training needs that GPStRs can incorporate into their Personal Development Plan (PDP).

Conducting a CbD: a worked example

Imagine your GPStR offers a case for CbD concerning a 67-year-old lady who is in the early stages of dementia. She lives alone in a sheltered housing flat. Her only daughter lives locally but is emigrating to Spain in the next month or so. The paperwork from the GPStR might look like this:

Reason for attendance: she is very itchy 'down below' and the nurse told her two months ago to see a doctor.

PMH:
depression
osteoarthritis
hypertension
hyperlipidaemia
Type 2 diabetes
CKD 3

Results (two months ago):
HbA1c 11.6, cholesterol 7.2, TG 8.6, eGFR 57

Medication:
avandamet 4/1000 bd
ramipril 10 mg om
atorvastatin 40 mg on
insulin
citalopram 20 mg om

Continued over

> **Consultation:**
> Says she feels well.
> Glad the diabetic nurse has stopped her insulin as she never got the hang of it.
> Hasn't done any home testing since she saw the nurse. c/o itch 'down below'
> o/e looks like candidal vulvitis with secondary excoriation.
> Denies missing any medication.
> Says she tries to eat a healthy diet but giggles about occasionally having cream buns as a treat.
> Records show numerous entries from the diabetic nurse discussing diet.
> Arranged blood test (HbA1, BG, P+E lipids).
> Asked to come back next week for review with the result.

STEP 1 ◊ before reading further take a moment to consider which competence areas are of relevance in this case.

There are probably seven relevant competences in this case:

  2 ◊ practising holistically
  3 ◊ data gathering and interpretation
  4 ◊ making a diagnosis/making decisions
  5 ◊ clinical management
  6 ◊ managing medical complexity and promoting health
  8 ◊ working with colleagues and in teams
 11 ◊ maintaining an ethical approach to practice.

STEP 2 ◊ select no more than three and, using a copy of the planning sheet, prepare some questions for each competence.

Selecting the competences depends on the situation, the GPStR's level of experience, what areas you have already assessed and what evidence you have so far about his or her ability. You may, for example, have had some evidence from multi-source feedback (MSF) that the GPStR needs to improve communications with the Primary Health Care Team (PHCT). You may have developed some concerns about his or her ability to manage complexity after a recent random case analysis or you may not yet have explored ethical issues at all.

For the purposes of this exercise let us assume that 6, 8 and 11 are the three competences you choose to discuss.

STEP 3 ◊ plan the questions you will use to guide the discussion (see Box 9.4).

BOX 9.4 **Planning the questions**	
Competence	**Proposed questions**
6 ☐ *Managing medical complexity and promoting health*	■ What was the patient's main concern? ■ What did you think her health problems were? ■ How did that affect your management? ■ What are the issues raised in this case? ■ What conflicts were you trying to resolve? ■ Why did you find it difficult/challenging?
8 ☐ *Working with colleagues and in teams*	■ Which colleagues did you involve in this case? Why? ■ How did you communicate with them? ■ Who could you have involved? What might they have been able to offer?
11 ☐ *Maintaining an ethical approach to practice*	■ What did you see as being the ethical problems in this case? ■ What ethical framework did you refer to in this case? How did you apply it? ■ How did it help you decide what to do? ■ How did you establish the patient's point of view? ■ What are her rights? How did this influence your handling of the case?

Clearly, in any discussion, questions are not delivered in isolation but will be tailored to the responses of the GPStR.

STEP 4 ◊ think carefully about what evidence you will be looking for in order to make a judgement about these competences and record this on the planning sheet (see Box 9.5).

BOX 9.5 **Looking for evidence**	
Competence	**Evidence to look for**
6 ☐ *Managing medical complexity and promoting health*	■ Does the doctor understand the difference between the doctor's understanding of the importance of the patient's multiple health problems and the things that concern the patient? ■ Does the doctor demonstrate an ability to manage the complexity of multiple pathology in a patient who does not appreciate its implications and has no motivation to change?
8 ☐ *Working with colleagues and in teams*	■ Does the doctor understand the benefits of teamwork in chronic disease management? ■ Is the suggested form of communication appropriate? ■ Does the doctor appreciate the important contribution of the diabetic nurse and what can be learnt from her experience?

Continued over

| 11 □ *Maintaining an ethical approach to practice* | ■ Does the doctor see any ethical issues?
■ Does the doctor have an ethical framework that helps him or her to deal with the problem?
■ Can the doctor apply an ethical framework appropriately? |

Grading judgement

This is an area that concerns most trainers when they are first introduced to CbD. It is important to keep returning to both word pictures (the developmental word pictures and the detailed competence descriptors) very regularly when making your judgement about the performance of the GPStR. Be reassured that MRCGP oral examiners, no matter how experienced they are and how well they have internalised the descriptors, still refer to both word pictures throughout the 20 minute oral examination while making their judgement.

Let us consider what evidence we might look for at each level of performance in this particular case (see Box 9.6).

BOX 9.6 Making judgements

6 □ Managing medical complexity and promoting health

Insufficient evidence	Needs further development	Competent	Excellent
Doesn't even recognise that there are a number of medical problems that require dealing with, e.g. may treat the consultation at face value and only treat the vulvitis	Is aware that there is more than one problem to deal with and that the consultation is complex	Quickly works out the patient's presenting complaint; this requires quick attention to allow plenty of time to discuss and agree a plan for the longer-term health issues	Works out an appropriate plan of action for how to deal with the patient's multiple pathology, which includes the doctor arranging a process to remind the patient when she is next due to come to surgery
	Deals with the patient's vulvitis first and then tackles the longer-term health issues Recognises that it will be difficult to achieve optimal care for this patient	Recognises that they can't all be dealt with in one consultation and regular review will be required	Recognises that whatever the patient says now, she may not remember or believe what you've asked her to do is important

	Recognises that this patient requires a lot of support and education	Helps the patient to understand that she needs to come back regularly	Manages to get her to prioritise what troubles her most and negotiates a plan for dealing with it that also allows the doctor to review her physical health

8 ☐ Working with colleagues and in teams

Insufficient evidence	Needs further development	Competent	Excellent
Hasn't even recognised the need to involve anyone else	Appropriately contacts the diabetic nurse to get more information about what happened two months ago and to arrange support for the patient	Arranges a meeting with the important parties to discuss the patient's ongoing care	Uses the patient's care and the team meeting to encourage others to use this event as a learning process
	Recognises the need to discuss her care with her daughter (with her permission) and the warden of the sheltered accommodation	Demonstrates a willingness to learn from other team members	

11 ☐ Maintaining an ethical approach to practice

Insufficient evidence	Needs further development	Competent	Excellent
Doesn't realise there is an ethical dimension to this case	Recognises that this is a tricky ethical case but may need prompting to recognise issues of competence, beneficence and non-maleficence (among others)	Manages to easily identity the ethical issues in the case and has already applied an ethical framework to help guide what to do	Understands that it may be necessary to accept that optimal care is not possible and can justify this by balancing ethical principles
	Demonstrates respect for this old lady and doesn't condescend or try to railroad her treatment without attempts at negotiation	Sensitively checks with the diabetic nurse what her attitude to this difficult case is to ensure that the patient's care has not been compromised by prejudice	

How the outcomes of CbD can inform future learning

In addition to the assessment process, your conclusions from the CbD and the conversation that this is likely to have provoked are likely to identify future learning needs. Some GPStRs may need prompting if they find this difficult. It is then important to help them to agree what specific actions they will take to address these needs.

Standard setting for CbD

When trainers are first introduced to CbD, one of their anxieties is how they will know the standard against which they are making judgements. This is largely because we are familiar with traditional summative and formative models of assessment but CbD requires a mind shift. It is not an examination and therefore there is no pass/fail level. Rather it is a process where evidence is collected and recorded. It is the accumulation of all the evidence collected by CbD, the other tools used in WPBA and naturally occurring evidence that will enable the trainer to judge whether the GPStR is progressing as one might expect or is failing to develop and therefore needs extra support.

CbDs should be conducted by more than one assessor during each period of training. The assessor must know how to conduct CbD but could be a registrar in the hospital setting or a neighbouring trainer. This will allow a wider interpretation of the GPStR's ability and progress, and is likely to help educators to feel supported with their assessment.

Just as all assessors should be trained and prepared for the task, there is also a need for ongoing development for assessors. Box 9.7 contains a few suggestions.

BOX 9.7 Suggestions for assessor development

- Use educational meetings or trainers' workshops to compare the experience of CbD with your colleagues.

- Try recording a CbD and then looking at it with other assessors, marking it as you go, before comparing your assessments and discussing the evidence underpinning your judgements.

- Sit in with other colleagues as they conduct a CbD. Discuss it afterwards with them. You will both learn from this process.

- Use the RCGP DVD workbook package *Talking the Talk*,[7] which shows examples of CbD on DVD with a supporting workbook (available from the College's Online Bookstore, www.rcgp.org.uk/acatalog).

- Practise doing CbDs in threes at your trainers' workshop or educational meetings.

REFERENCES

1. Schuwirth LWT, Southgate L, Page GG, *et al.* When enough is enough: a conceptual basis for fair and defensible practice performance assessment *Medical Education* 2002; 36(10): 925–30.

2. Jannett PA, Affleck L. Chart audit and chart stimulated recall as methods of needs assessment in continuing professional health education *Journal of Continuing Education in the Health Professions* 1998; 18: 163–71.

3. Accreditation Council for Graduate Medical Education. *ACGME Outcomes Project: toolbox of assessment methods* Evanston, Illinois: American Board of Medical Specialties, 2000.

4. Wakeford R, Southgate L, Wass V. Improving oral examinations: selecting, training, and monitoring examiners for the MRCGP *British Medical Journal* 1995; 311(7010): 931–5.

5. Wass V, Wakeford R, Neighbour R, *et al.* Achieving acceptable reliability in oral examinations: an analysis of the Royal College of General Practitioners membership examination's oral component *Medical Education* 2003; 37: 126–31.

6. Elstein AS. Beyond multiple-choice questions and essays: the need for a new way to assess clinical competence *Academic Medicine* 1993; 68(4): 244–9.

7. Chana N, Gardiner P, Rughani A, *et al. Talking the Talk: using case-based discussion in medical assessments* London: RCGP, 2007.

8. Department of Health. *Modernising Medical Careers: the next steps* London: DH, 2007.

9. Department of Health. *Modernising Medical Careers* London: DH, 2007, www.mmc.nhs.uk/pages/assessment/cbd [accessed December 2007].

10. Southgate L, Cox J, David T, *et al.* The assessment of poorly performing doctors: the development of the assessment programmes for the GMC's performance procedures *Medical Education* 2001; 35: 2–8.

11. Southgate L, Cox J, David T, *et al.* The General Medical Council's performance procedures: the development and implementation of tests of competence with examples from general practice *Medical Education* 2001; 35: 20 8.

12. Joughin G. Dimensions of oral assessment *Assessment and Evaluation in Higher Education* 1998; 23: 367–78.

13. Joughin G. Dimensions of oral assessment and student approaches to learning. In: S Brown, A Glasner (eds). *Assessment Matters*, pp. 146–56, Buckingham: The Society for Research into Higher Education and the Open University Press, 1999.

14. Joughin G, Collom G. *Oral Assessment* York: Higher Education Academy, 2004, www.heacademy.ac.uk/assets/York/documents/resources/resourcedatabase/id433_oral_assessment.pdf [accessed December 2007].

15. Finucane P, Gisele A, Boureois-Law M, *et al.* Comparison or performance assessment systems in Canada, Australia, New Zealand and the UK *Academic Medicine* 2003; 78: 837–43.

16. Cunnington J, Hanna E, Turnbull J, *et al.* Defensible assessment of the competency of the practicing physician *Academic Medicine* 1997; 72: 9–12.

17. Royal College of General Practitioners. *A Brief Guide to Workplace Based Assessment in the nMRCGP* London: RCGP, 2007, www.rcgp.org.uk/docs/nMRCGP_WPBA_in_the_nMRCGP_sep07.doc [accessed December 2007].

101

10 Workplace-Based Assessment

The consultation observation tool

Mei Ling Denney and Mark Coombe

The consultation observation tool (COT) is one of a number of assessment tools that have been designed to collect evidence to support the holistic judgements that have to be made about GPStRs during their training. In hospital placements, the mini-clinical evaluation exercise (mini-CEX) tool is also used, which does not require video-recorded patient encounters. However, the starting point for the COT can be either a video-recorded consultation or a directly observed consultation by the trainer. In either case the observation should generate discussion and feedback for the GPStR.

If we include a timetable as to what needs to be achieved and when for the WPBA during training, this does not future-proof this book in case of RCGP changes. For a timetable of which Workplace-Based Assessment (WPBA) tools need to be completed and when, see www.rcgp.org.uk/the_gp_journey/nmrcgp/wpba_and_eportfolio/collecting_evidence.aspx.

The ability to create and maintain effective doctor–patient relationships is an essential quality for any doctor. Consulting skills are an important part of a doctor's continuing professional development, and similar videotaped assessments have been used in reviews of performance later in a GP's career.[1]

Introduced in 1996, the consulting skills module of the examination for membership of the Royal College of General Practitioners (MRCGP) resulted in registrars devoting time and effort towards improving their consultation skills. Whilst not appropriate for every consultation, the ability to demonstrate patient-centredness is held by the RCGP to be a marker of good general practice. Evidence shows that training healthcare providers in patient-centred approaches may impact positively on patient satisfaction with their care.[2]

The COT has developed from the MRCGP video performance criteria. These criteria were developed following a wide literature search and subsequently modified by consultation with over a hundred practising general practitioners, thus giving good content validity.[3]

Videotape review has been found by researchers elsewhere to have similar validity and reliability to direct observation.[4] However, there are also significant threats to validity associated with authenticity, generalisability, domain definition and sampling.[5] With fewer consultations, these problems are magnified.

Reliability issues in the MRCGP video exam were addressed by initial and ongoing training of examiners, double-marking exercises, detailed discussions around the performance criteria, and personalised feedback to examiners. It was enhanced by the close working of examiners, with continuity maintained by low examiner turnover. These principles will need to be embraced by trainer groups, and the organisations that support them.

The MRCGP video module fell short of a complete performance assessment because the candidates selected consultations to represent their 'best' efforts. The issue of representativeness was also raised by the paucity of high-challenge cases seen in candidates' video submissions. To achieve a 'generalisable' result, a large number of skills and content topics need to be sampled. For the COT, at least 12 cases should be observed and judged by the trainer, as this amount of time on assessment of video-recorded consultations has been shown to give acceptable levels of reliability, as well as being considered acceptable by both GPs and patients.[4]

The COT differs from the video submission in several important ways:

- GPStRs no longer submit a tape to be assessed by external examiners from the College; the trainer is now the assessor
- trainers will grade their registrars on each performance criterion, and make a global judgement on each consultation
- the emphasis of the COT is formative; registrars will not 'fail'. Instead, the evidence collected from each consultation will inform the overall process and feed into training
- the performance criteria have changed, and there are no 'merit' criteria.

The video exam has sometimes been criticised for placing too little emphasis on clinical skills. The performance criteria have therefore been revised for the COT to allow a shift of emphasis towards the assessment of clinical skills.

TIPS

□ The RCGP website is a valuable source of information that needs to be checked regularly in order to be aware of any new guidance or revisions to the COT (www.rcgp.org.uk/the_gp_journey/nmrcgp/wpba_tools/cot.aspx).

□ Trainers should share views and experiences within trainers' workshops so that a consistent approach is possible.

How does the COT relate to the e-portfolio?

The COT provides an opportunity for evidence to be gathered under most of the 12 units of competence detailed in the e-portfolio. Five of these are particularly relevant to the COT:

- communication and consultation skills
- practising holistically

- data gathering and interpretation
- making a diagnosis/making decisions
- clinical management.

Carrying out a COT

Two consultations should normally be viewed for in-training assessment purposes at each sitting. For details on frequency and timing of COTs during training, see the College website.

Immediately after each observation of any video-recorded or live consultation, the trainer will enter his or her grades and comments directly into the COT section of the e-portfolio, including notes for formative feedback and suggestions for further development. The registrar will be able to see both that the assessment has been completed, and all the comments that have been added. Once submitted, it will not be possible to alter or remove the record of a particular COT.

TIPS

□ Both GPStRs and trainers should familiarise themselves thoroughly with the e-portfolio units of competence.

□ It is a good idea to get into the habit of documenting specific examples of evidence of competence in the portfolio, as it arises and is seen during COT assessments, as well as submitting the COTs themselves.

What can be done to prepare?

As part of their training in and for general practice, GPStRs have daily opportunities to learn and improve on communication and clinical skills. This includes encounters with patients in regular and emergency surgeries during the day, home visits, and out-of-hours practice. It is helpful to record consultations on video, so that these can be observed and reflected on by the registrar and, most importantly, can be shared with others in order for the learner to benefit from constructive feedback. This process should start as soon as is practically possible during general practice placements, and should not be seen simply as last-minute preparation for the COT.

Other ways of preparing include:

- being familiar with the content of the RCGP curriculum statements for training, and the exam syllabus
- using books and other training materials on consultation skills; trying out, and becoming confident in, at least one of the consultation models

■ observing others in consultations, by sitting in with trainers and other GPs, or by sharing learning by viewing other GPStRs' consultations in learner sets.

TIP

□ Think of questions to ask the patient that may reveal his or her agenda or health beliefs, e.g. 'How is this illness affecting your work/home/school/life?' 'What were you worried about?' 'What were you hoping I would do?'

If the consultation for the COT is to be recorded for subsequent viewing, it is important to consider sound and vision quality – if these are poor, the consultation will be difficult for the trainer to assess accurately. If the consultation is to be directly observed, attention should be paid to the consulting room that will be used. This should have enough space for an observer to be present without being obtrusive. All consultations must be conducted either in English or in another language common to patient, GPStR and trainer/assessor.

TIPS

□ Build up a good base of general practice-related knowledge, and become familiar with at least one of the consultation models.

□ Get to grips with recording technology, to be able to produce good-quality recordings.

□ Start recording consultations on video or DVD as early on as possible, and share these with others in the training arena to guide learning.

□ Arrange joint consultations with your trainer, to observe another GP's consulting skills, and to be comfortable with another person sitting in on your own consultation with a patient.

What kind of consultations should be selected?

Registrars may either record a number of consultations on video and select one for assessment and discussion, or agree prospectively with the trainer to choose one patient encounter that will be the subject of direct observation. In either case the GPStR must ensure that the patient has given consent as per the RCGP guidelines. To give their informed consent, patients must be able to understand the purpose of the recording or observation, and must not be coerced into agreeing to have their consultation recorded or watched.

Over the entire period of training spent in general practice, at least one case from each of the following categories should be included:

- children (aged 10 or under)
- older adults (an adult aged more than 75 years' old)
- patients with mental health problems.

Up to two consultations may be viewed for in-training assessment purposes on each occasion.

A wide variety of consultations is more likely to offer the GP registrar the opportunity to demonstrate the full range of competences. It would be best to avoid the temptation of selecting very low-challenge consultations for the COT, as this strategy will neither allow the doctor to meet many of the performance criteria, nor provide the insights that he or she will need for improvement in consultation skills, and preparation for external assessment in the form of the Clinical Skills Assessment (CSA).

107

As a general rule, it is inadvisable for a consultation to exceed more than 15 minutes in duration, unless there is good reason, as effective use of time is taken into account when considering the performance criterion on 'resources'. Complex consultations, or those containing a strong psychological aspect, are more likely to justify greater consultation length. GPStRs towards the end of their training would be expected to make more effective use of time than those at the start of their experience in general practice.

It is not usually possible to demonstrate all competences within a single consultation, and GPStRs are strongly advised not to attempt to do so, as this may lend the consultation artificiality, and result in undesirable and unhelpful mechanistic behaviours.

TIPS

□ Choose a wide variety of consultations, including straightforward or more complex conditions, and patients with acute or chronic illnesses.

□ Include consultations with a clear clinical component, as well as those with a clear psychosocial component.

□ Consultations with greater complexity are an opportunity to generate more evidence for the assessment, and produce more useful formative feedback.

□ Restrict the number of follow-up appointments, as these are less likely to give the doctor an opportunity to demonstrate meeting the performance criteria, compared with those where the patient is consulting for his or her condition for the first time.

What is acceptable during a COT consultation?

GPStRs and trainers may be anxious about the acceptability of parts of the consultation when performed for the COT. This may include clinical examination, and use of resources within the consultation.

For recorded consultations, it is quite acceptable to perform simple examinations such as taking a patient's blood pressure or an ear, nose or throat examination 'on camera', but any potentially embarrassing physical examinations are best done off camera, with the sound recorded if possible so that any conversation between the doctor and the patient can still be heard. Patients are more likely to give consent to be video-recorded if their dignity is preserved. For observed consultations, the acceptability of the trainer watching the clinical part of the consultation is likely to be higher, particularly if the trainer is known to the patient. Nevertheless, the patient's consent for this should be explicit.

As for non-observed consultations, the GPStR should have access to all the usual sources of information. This will include the computerised and written patient records, internet sources of information such as guidelines and protocols, reference books and clinical formularies. Referring to sources of information (including asking advice from a colleague) will, however, eat into the consultation time, and may be taken into account under 'use of resources'.

Relationships with patients in general practice are longitudinal, and continuity of care is valued by patients. It is not necessary to complete the diagnosis and management of the patient in one consultation, but it is important to demonstrate that they have made an appropriate differential diagnosis, and a management plan that includes follow-up if necessary.

What are the units of competence and performance criteria for the COT?

There are five units of competence from the nMRCGP e-portfolio that can be addressed by COT:

- discover the reason for the patient's attendance
- define the clinical problem(s)
- explain the problem(s) to the patient
- address the patient's problem(s)
- make effective use of the consultation.

The COT performance criteria can be divided into:

- those that require demonstration of active listening skills
- those that can sometimes be satisfied by a purely doctor-centred approach
- those that specifically require patient-centred skills with active involvement of the patient, particularly in management of patient problems.

Candidates who actively listen, display an interest in their patients as people, show clinical competence and attempt to involve their patients in the decision-making process are generally more likely to achieve an 'Excellent' grade.

Box 10.1 contains a list of the performance criteria that the GPStR is required to demonstrate. Commentaries on each can be found on the RCGP website or within the e-portfolio.

BOX 10.1 **COT performance criteria**

1 ☐ The doctor is seen to encourage the patient's contribution at appropriate points in the consultation.

2 ☐ The doctor is seen to respond to signals (cues) that lead to a deeper understanding of the problem.

3 ☐ The doctor uses appropriate psychological and social information to place the complaint(s) in context.

4 ☐ The doctor explores the patient's health understanding.

5 ☐ The doctor obtains sufficient information to include or exclude likely relevant significant conditions.

6 ☐ The physical/mental examination chosen is likely to confirm or disprove hypotheses that could reasonably have been formed, or is designed to address a patient's concern.

7 ☐ The doctor appears to make a clinically appropriate working diagnosis.

8 ☐ The doctor explains the problem or diagnosis in appropriate language.

9 ☐ The doctor specifically seeks to confirm the patient's understanding of the diagnosis.

10 ☐ The management plan (including any prescription) is appropriate for the working diagnosis, reflecting a good understanding of modern accepted medical practice.

11 ☐ The patient is given the opportunity to be involved in significant management decisions.

12 ☐ Makes effective use of resources.

13 ☐ The doctor specifies the conditions and interval for follow-up or review.

How is the COT consultation assessed?

Whilst the trainer may well conduct the majority of these assessments, it is recommended that at least one other assessor is involved in judging a few of the COTs. This could be another trainer within the practice, a trainer outside the practice, or a course organiser (training/programme director). This will enable objective judgements to be made by more than one person, and a different perspective to be obtained, giving the potential for more useful formative feedback.

During the COT session, the trainer grades each of the items as:

(1) INSUFFICIENT EVIDENCE
From the available evidence, the doctor's performance cannot be placed on a higher point of this developmental scale. This should not be taken to be a 'bad fail', but rather may be a consequence of selecting a consultation that simply did not lend itself to demonstrating that particular competence.

(N) NEEDS FURTHER DEVELOPMENT

The GPStR demonstrates a rigid adherence to taught rules or plans and has a superficial grasp of unconnected facts. He or she is unable to apply knowledge and has little situational perception or discretionary judgement.

(C) COMPETENT

110

The GPStR accesses and applies coherent and appropriate chunks of knowledge. He or she is able to see actions with regards to longer-term goals, can demonstrate conscious and deliberate planning with increased level of efficiency, can cope with crowdedness and is able to prioritise.

(E) EXCELLENT

The GPStR has an intuitive and holistic grasp of situations, no longer relying on rules or maxims. He or she can identify underlying principles and patterns to define and solve problems, can relate recalled information to the goals of the present situation, and is aware of the conditions for application of that knowledge.

It is worth noting that it may be unrealistic to expect doctors at an early stage of their careers to demonstrate all the skills sought by trainers. Towards the start of training in general practice, it is likely that many of the grades will be 'N'. This is not to be seen as unexpected, as a key aspect is that the COT provides information on which further teaching and learning can be based. It is anticipated, however, that as the registrar spends further time in training there should be a shift from the 'N' to the 'C' grades. If this is not the case, the registrar is unlikely to do well in the nMRCGP CSA, and needs further feedback and targeted training.

Trainers should consider the expected standard of a GP registrar at the end point of GP specialty training when making their judgements, and not expect a performance similar to that of an experienced GP.

Currently the assessor is asked to make a single global judgement on the whole consultation viewed. However, there is evidence to suggest that performance criteria 2, 3, 4, 9, 11 and 13 assess consulting skills and 5, 6, 7, 8, 10 and 11 assess clinical skills. It is quite possible that in the future trainers may be asked to award two global ratings to reflect these two aspects.

TIPS

☐ Adequate protected time must be allowed for during the COT assessment.

☐ Trainers and registrars should plan to include at least one other assessor other than the usual trainer for the COT.

☐ Agreement about the expected standard should be reached between trainers in a trainer group, relating this to national standards.

☐ The meaning of the *I, N, C* and *E* grades should be discussed and understood in training sessions for both trainers and registrars.

☐ Performance in the COT consultations can serve as a guide to the state of preparedness of registrars to undertake the CSA.

REFERENCES   111

1. Norman G, Davis D, Lamb S, *et al*. Competency assessment of primary care physicians as part of a peer review program *Journal of the American Medical Association* 1993; 270(9): 1046.

2. Lewin SA, Skea ZC, Entwistle V, *et al*. Interventions for providers to promote a patient-centred approach in clinical consultations *Cochrane Database of Systematic Reviews* 2001; 4: CD003267.

3. Tate P, Foulkes J, Neighbour R, *et al*. Assessing physicians' interpersonal skills via videotaped encounters: a new approach for the MRCGP *Journal of Health Communication* 1999; 4: 143–52.

4. Ram P, Grol R, Rethans JJ, *et al*. Assessment of general practitioners by video observation in daily practice: issues of validity, reliability and feasibility *Medical Education* 1999; 33: 447–54.

5. Swanwick T. The video component of the MRCGP examination: threats to validity *Education for Primary Care* 2004; 15(3): 311–27.

11   The Clinical Skills Assessment process

Amar Rughani

Clinical Skills Assessment (CSA) is an OSCE-style examination and is one of the three components of the MRCGP. Its objective is to assess the doctor's ability to integrate and apply appropriate clinical, professional, communication and practical skills in general practice. Although these skills are routinely witnessed in the workplace, the CSA can test them reliably by using simulated patients and testing in standardised contexts to a predetermined level of challenge. Although a CSA circuit of cases cannot systematically test everything that happens in the workplace, it can 'spot check', using a selection of cases drawn from across the curriculum.

Assessors are not looking for rare, esoteric or complicated skills that are seldom used in real life. Quite the opposite. The standard to pass is not the standard that might be expected from experienced GPs but of GPs who are new to independent practice and therefore need to be competent in dealing with a patient's problems without the need for supervision.

Let's have a quick walk through the exam.

The exam mimics a GP surgery and therefore the doctor stays in the consulting room whilst at intervals a series of simulated patients, expertly played by actors, present their problems. The consultations are ten minutes' long and there is a short, approximately two-minute, break between them. Each actor is accompanied by an assessor and the duo of patient/assessor move around the circuit of candidates portraying the same case in a standardised way to each candidate. The role-player takes no part in making the formal assessment of candidate performance.

Although 13 patients are seen, one of the cases will be a pilot of a new case and will not count toward the candidate's overall mark. The candidate will not be made aware which of the 13 cases is the pilot.

BOX 11.1 **Practical considerations**

The CSA examination can only be attempted in ST3, the final year of training, or within 12 months of the expected date of completion of training.

Only three attempts are allowed. Unsuccessful candidates will need to discuss the outcomes with their area programme director or head of school.

Candidates are required to bring to the CSA their normal doctor's bag, with a BNF. The

Continued over

> specific equipment required will be notified to candidates in good time before they attend for their assessment. The mock consulting room will have basic equipment.
>
> For costs and application process, please see the RCGP website (www.rcgp.org.uk/the_gp_journey/nmrcgp/csa.aspx).

The cases

At the heart of CSA are the cases and these are written by assessors who are all experienced and practising GPs. The cases are designed to test different areas of the GP curriculum and are often informed by real-life situations, making them representative of contemporary British general practice.

A case selection blueprint is used to select the cases in the circuit. This ensures that:

- VARIOUS CLINICAL CONTEXTS ◊ such as cardiovascular, endocrine, psychiatric, etc., are tested
- VARIOUS TYPES OF ENCOUNTER ◊ such as acute or chronic presentations, are seen
- VARIOUS TYPES OF PATIENT ◊ such as children, the elderly, patients from different social and cultural backgrounds, etc., are included in the mix.

In addition, the cases are changed daily. As we can see, this is a complex affair!

TIP

CSA comprises a number of cases that are constructed based on several factors. Examples that illustrate different types of cases and an explanation of how these cases are derived can be seen on the RCGP website (www.rcgp.org.uk/the_gp_journey/nmrcgp/csa.aspx).

Each case is accompanied by instructions to the role-player, instructions to the assessor, the doctor's case notes and the case-specific marking schedule. Candidates will only see the case notes, of course.

These case notes are constructed to look as similar to medical case notes as possible, although they are not in electronic form. Only the relevant details are presented, including significant past medical history, current medication, social habits, etc. The patient's last consultation may also be available, or a relevant letter from secondary care, test results, ECGs, etc. The case notes are kept to the essential minimum so that candidates do not have to wade through unnecessary details to learn about their 'patients'.

The final and most important part of the case is the marking schedule. This has been carefully tailored to the assessment purpose of the case and the following broad areas, or 'domains', are assessed in each of the cases:

- information gathering
- clinical management
- interpersonal skills.

In the marking schedule, guidance is provided to assessors as to what to look for in terms of appropriate or inappropriate behaviour in the given situation. Assessors use this guidance and their observations to mark each domain separately and then, based on this, produce an 'overall' grade for the case. There are four possible grades, which are:

- clear pass
- marginal pass
- marginal fail
- clear fail.

The candidate needs to pass a certain number of cases to pass the assessment overall and each candidate is sent feedback on his or her performance in the CSA as well as his or her marks. This feedback contains both positive and negative comments on the candidate's performance, and is intended to help candidates gain a greater educational insight into their performance.

TIPS

It is only natural that candidates would try to prepare strategically for the CSA, but, as we have seen, the case writing and case selection processes are complex. Even if trainees found out from previous candidates about the cases they had seen, they would not be able to second-guess what the assessor was looking for.

It is far better for GPStRs to approach each case as they would a new patient in surgery. This will keep minds open and alert, and stop them from going down the wrong route. The key message is: 'Focus on the patient, not what you imagine the assessor is looking for.'

Candidates will be sent feedback based on their performance. The advice that forms the basis of this feedback is available from the RCGP website and is a useful resource in helping all candidates to prepare, whether they have taken the exam or not.

What is CSA testing for?

The MRCGP is designed to test the learning outcomes stated in the GP curriculum. The curriculum is available on the RCGP website (www.rcgp-curriculum. org.uk).

TIPS

Obtain the curriculum statements from the RCGP website and read through them thoroughly. Most curriculum statements have a section on 'common and important conditions' and CSA cases are quite likely to be based on these.

The curriculum statements are regularly updated, so learners should make sure they have the most recent versions.

The curriculum has six core competences:

- primary care management
- person-centred care
- specific problem-solving skills
- a comprehensive approach
- community orientation
- a holistic approach.

The CSA is designed to test the first three of these, which together form the basis of the patient-centred clinical method.[1] These skills are at the heart of the primary care consultation and are shown in Figure 11.1.

FIGURE 11.1 The patient-centred clinical method [1,2]

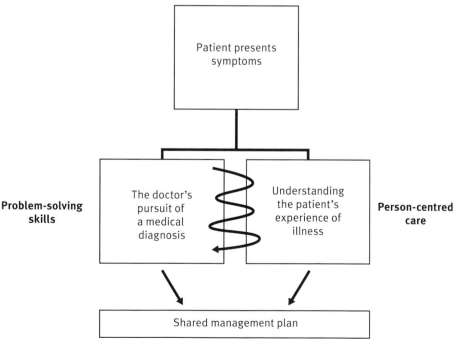

Figure 11.1 shows how the doctor uses biomedical problem-solving skills that are gained through years of medical training. In addition to this, the doctor uses communication skills to listen, explore the patient's thoughts, understand the context of the problem in relation to the patient's life and negotiate an appropriate management plan.

In an adept consultation, these two strands are tightly interwoven. Mastering these competences and thereby demonstrating the patient-centred clinical method is the key to success in the exam.

The remaining three core competences of the curriculum are touched upon in CSA, and may form part of a case, but they are not the prime focus.

TIPS

The best way to prepare for CSA is to concentrate on what goes on in the consulting room and to practise the patient-centred clinical method until this becomes fluent.

Assessors will only know whether or not the candidate has *good biomedical skills* if they hear medical issues being discussed. These include the likely diagnoses, an assessment of risk, and the appropriate management options.

Assessors will reward a *patient-centred approach* when they see candidates try to understand how the problem relates to the patient's life and by the way they share and negotiate during the consultation, particularly regarding the management plan.

Assessors will pick up on *interpersonal skills* through the doctor's demeanour and communication skills.

A broader understanding of primary care beyond the consulting room is important, but is not the focus of CSA.

How can we help learners develop their clinical skills for CSA?

In everyday practice, doctors apply their clinical skills through the following continuum:

gathering data from selective history/examination/investigation, including the use of instruments

interpreting the results of these data and deciding upon their significance

creating a hypothesis ('What might be the problem?')

↓

formulating/justifying a diagnosis and management plan

↓

monitoring/reviewing and learning from the outcomes.

In CSA, learners must demonstrate that their approach is:

- consistent with current accepted medical practice, for example by developing management plans that are evidence based and in line with nationally accepted guidelines
- systematic and appropriately selective
- efficient, with good time management.
- proficient, with respect to the ability to perform the examinations and use diagnostic and therapeutic instruments of the type commonly used by GPs.

Many elements of the continuum shown above can be tested in the Clinical Skills Assessment. Let us look at these in more detail.

Gathering data from selective history/examination/investigations

This requires learners to be appropriately selective in the questions they ask, the tests they request and the examinations they choose to undertake. Learners may feel that it would be better to be 'on the safe side' by ordering a battery of tests and, whilst understandable, this is not good practice and will make them appear indiscriminate, disorganised and wasteful of resources. Likewise, history taking and examination are not expected to be all-inclusive and should be tailored to the circumstances.

Being selective requires learners to demonstrate that they understand what is likely, what is less likely and what is unlikely but important. Learners should first ensure that their knowledge base is up to scratch and then improve their skills by sharing their thoughts with the patient. For example, they might explain what they are looking for, what they think the likely diagnosis might be and (where appropriate) what they feel is unlikely but needs to be ruled out.

TIPS

Educators can help develop these skills by first encouraging learners to develop an appropriate mindset. Try exploring the learner's understanding, attitudes and motivation by asking about:

- □ the downside of a scattergun approach to data gathering
- □ the benefits to the patient of targeted questioning and investigation
- □ the benefits to society of being selective
- □ how to achieve a balance between gathering information and minimising risk.

Assessors need to see that the candidate has a rational and justifiable approach. As educators, we can help learners to achieve this by encouraging them to explain to the patient what they are proposing to do and why. As well as being good for exam preparation, this behaviour is also good for patient care.

Performing examinations and using instruments proficiently

Improving these skills is a matter of practice and it pays for learners to spend time developing a systematic method that can be practised repeatedly. Before doing so, educators can help by checking that the technique is correct so that learners are not simply reinforcing bad habits. Once correct techniques are practised and become fluent, the approach will appear competent and confident to the assessor.

TIPS

Think about the common types of clinical examination that are seen in everyday general practice and then encourage learners to practise focused examinations. Educators can observe and give feedback. There are some examinations that are very unlikely to be tested, for example intimate examinations, but candidates could be asked to assess a leg, arm, chest, abdomen, etc.

Make sure that candidates are conversant with any medical equipment that might be needed, and can handle it with confidence.

Interpreting the results of these data and deciding upon their significance

Candidates might be asked to interpret the significance of test results or the findings of physical and mental state examinations. These will nearly always relate to common or important conditions. The data may be given to the candidate before the consultation or may arise during the consultation. For example, the candidate may request to perform a particular examination and in some situations would be given the results of such an examination by the assessor. Deciding upon 'significance' often means demonstrating that risk has been assessed and priorities appropriately determined.

TIPS

Encourage learners to think about the sort of letters they receive from secondary care and the types of test results they see (ECGs, spirometry, blood test results, urinalysis results, skin scrapings, swabs, smear results, etc.).

Ask what they make of them, the urgency with which they should be attended to and how the results might be explained to the patient.

Encourage learners to discuss clinical management with colleagues, asking them particularly to share their experience of risk management and safety-netting.

Get learners to take an active part in significant event reviews (SEAs). Look back on SEAs relating to clinical errors and summarise what can be learnt.

Formulating/justifying a diagnosis and management plan

Although it may look like an ordinary surgery, CSA is different in important ways. As we might expect, candidates are unable to ask a colleague for a second opinion! More subtly, they do not have access to the usual sources of information, particularly the full patient records, internet sources of guidelines, etc., upon which most clinicians depend. Candidates will not be able to see the patient again, which means that they need to grasp the issue rather than defer, only deferring if it seems the appropriate thing to do in the circumstances.

Making a diagnosis means committing ourselves on the basis of the information that is available. Often, this may be a working diagnosis rather than one that is firmly established. The CSA case may not always require candidates to make a diagnosis, but, where this seems appropriate, common conditions should be considered in the differential diagnosis.

Candidates should ensure that their knowledge base is adequate as this is the foundation of clinical decision making. As educators, our role may include:

☐ reinforcing the importance of having knowledge, e.g. by testing the relevant knowledge base during the debrief and case-based discussion
☐ helping the learner to identify significant gaps.

When observing learners consult, we should make sure that, when a diagnosis is made, the doctor states this clearly and explains it to the patient using appropriate language. In the exam, if the summary is too vague, the assessor may not have sufficiently explicit evidence to be sure that the doctor has made a diagnosis at all.

The *management plan* needs to be in line with currently accepted practice and tailored to the patient's situation. The possible risks and benefits of different management approaches, including prescribing, need to be clearly identified and discussed with the patient. However, GPs are not simply there to inform the patient. Although patient autonomy is encouraged, candidates will be expected to assist the patient in making a decision by providing guidance based on their assessment of the situation.

Another and broader aspect of management is thinking about the prevention of future health-related problems. Health promotion requires candidates to demonstrate an awareness of health (rather than just illness) and to be proactive in maintaining the patient's health.

Hitherto in examinations of consulting skills, candidates have often shared management plans in simplistic and inappropriate ways, for example by providing a list of alternatives and leaving patients to take their pick from these with very little guidance.

As educators, we can help learners to share the management plan appropriately in terms of when to share, how much to discuss and how much to influence the shared decision.

Learners may not wish to share everything that they are thinking, perhaps because there would be little time for anything else or because they do not wish to alarm the patient. It is quite justified to be selective in what is said, but the key point is to get into the habit of sharing thoughts aloud with the patient and providing them with good explanations.

Learning to share in this way will lead to more effective and more time-efficient consultations.

In consultation, encourage learners to get into the habit of thinking 'How can I help my patient to remain well in the longer term and prevent ill-health from occurring prematurely?'

This mindset will automatically suggest which health promotion approaches might be appropriate. In addition, raising this issue with patients can help to empower them and take more control over their health.

Management plans will include arrangements for follow-up. These should reflect the natural history of the condition, be appropriate to the level of risk and be coherent and feasible.

How can we help learners develop their interpersonal skills for CSA?

Interpersonal skills are a combination of communication skills and attitudinal approaches to the patient. An effective method of developing *communication skills* is through observing learners consult, either on video or by 'sitting in', and then assessing them informally or more formally through a consultation observation tool (COT).

TIPS

Interpersonal skills lie at the heart of patient-centred consulting. A number of educational resources, particularly consulting skills books and videos, will help learners to understand the concept. We should encourage learners to have their performance assessed by colleagues, commenting in particular on:

☐ the doctor's ability to actively listen

☐ involving the patient and making use of verbal and non-verbal cues

☐ establishing the patient's agenda, health beliefs and preferences.

The main outcome of the patient-centred clinical method that was described earlier is the shared management plan. Assessors will look closely at how the doctor uses interpersonal skills to help patients develop this plan.

TIPS

The shared management plan may be improved by responding appropriately to the patient's agenda and by attempting to involve patients in making decisions regarding their problem. Educators should look closely at this behaviour when watching learners consult.

Clarifying the respective roles may involve reaching agreement with the patient as to what will happen next, who does what and when, and the conditions (i.e. the timescale and circumstances) for follow-up.

Explanations are essential to good-quality clinical care. They help patients to understand and to be sufficiently informed to make decisions. Exactly the same can be said for CSA assessors in the sense that they can't mark what they don't hear. Good explanations at all stages of the consultation will help the assessor to understand what the doctor is thinking and make an informed judgement – hopefully in the candidate's favour!

123

TIPS

In developing this skill, it is important for learners to avoid the use of jargon, to establish the patient's health beliefs and tailor their explanation to these.

Whether or not the explanation has been understood can be checked through non-verbal communication but also (and more explicitly) by asking the patient to summarise.

Attitudinal skills are concerned with the human dimension and the ability to take an active interest in the patient, treat him or her with respect, avoid prejudice, be aware of ethical issues and address these appropriately. It is likely that at least one of the cases in the circuit will test the ability to deal with issues related to diversity.

TIPS

These facets are not simply a matter of personality but are behaviours that can be taught. We can help learners to recognise and improve their attitudinal approach by probing what they learn about themselves from multi-source feedback from colleagues and from patient satisfaction questionnaires.

How do we assist learners to combine their clinical and interpersonal skills for CSA?

Get learners to video-record their consultations and watch them with a colleague, bearing in mind the points made above about the integration of clinical approach and interpersonal skills. The consultations could be marked for each of the two skills, and then for the combination of both. This would highlight the gaps in performance and therefore where the doctor should be working to improve.

Being able to combine the two areas in each consultation is vital, and comes with practice and with feedback so that it can be done not just in the occasional consultation, but in *every* consultation.

The final aspect of preparing for the CSA is the ability to cover all three domains (data gathering, clinical management and interpersonal skills) within a ten-minute consultation. The cases have been designed to be feasible to complete within the ten-minute slots, although to do this candidates will need to be efficient, organised and have a fluent approach. This seems a tall order, but candidates will not have to enter their consultations on computer or face some of the other interruptions that are common in surgery. Despite this, candidates who are slow consulters will find it difficult to finish a case in this time, and in their preparation they need to work on becoming time-efficient and focused. This is an aspect of training that may need particular attention.

124

TIPS

Think of the surgery consultations as 'mock CSAs'.

Assessing the consultation through the COT is an ideal way to judge readiness for the exam as it lends itself to more specific feedback.

It would be best not to select very low-challenge consultations for COT, tempting though this may be, as these will not give the insights that learners need for their preparation.

Learners need to show that they can *combine* good clinical skills with good interpersonal skills. Demonstrating clinical skills is often a matter of sharing thoughts with, and explaining effectively to, the patient.

As educators, we also can assist learners in practical ways by using the sample case material available from the RCGP website and setting up 'mock CSA' events in our localities.

REFERENCES

1. Levenstein JH, Belle Brown J, Weston WW, *et al*. Patient-centred clinical interviewing. In: M Stewart and D Roter (eds). *Communicating with Medical Patients* Newbury Park, CA: Sage Publications, 1989.

2. Stewart M, Brown J, Weston W, *et al*. *Patient-Centred Medicine: transforming the clinical method* Oxford: Radcliffe Medical Press, 2003.

12 The Applied Knowledge Test

Kay Mohanna

This chapter contains information taken from the RCGP website, www.rcgp.org.uk, in September 2007. All those planning to sit nMRCGP, or guiding others preparing for it, are advised to regularly check on the website for updates and advice about the exam.

The Applied Knowledge Test (AKT) is a summative assessment of the knowledge base that underpins independent general practice in the United Kingdom within the context of the National Health Service. Candidates who pass this assessment will have demonstrated their competence in applying knowledge at a level that is sufficiently high for independent practice.

Whilst candidates will be eligible to attempt the AKT at any point during their time in GP specialty training, it is anticipated that the most appropriate point, and that providing the highest chance of success, will be whilst working as a GPStR in the final year of their specialty training programme (ST3). A pass on this paper can be carried forward for three years, after which time it will need to be taken again if training has not been completed.

The test takes the form of a three-hour multiple-choice paper of 200 items. It is computer based and delivered at 150 professional testing centres around the UK, the same centres that administer the multiple-choice component of the driving test and the medical school selection processes. Candidates sit the test at a computer workstation, using a mouse and keyboard to select their answers. Before the test begins, candidates complete a brief tutorial on screen to ensure that they know how to record their answers and scroll through the questions.

We are all familiar with multiple-choice exams, having spent many hours sitting them or preparing for them over the years. But writing a good paper is not easy. In a classical multiple-choice question the learner should choose a correct answer among several (optimally five) answers. Multiple-choice questions consist of three obligatory parts, the question, the answer (or 'key') and several incorrect alternatives or distracters. The distracters should not give clues to the key or enable the answer to be correctly guessed.

A good multiple-choice paper examines only the important knowledge. Interesting small print or esoteric knowledge should not be included. Questions should be written in simple language, taking care with spelling and grammar to avoid ambiguity or confusion. In particular the text of the question should be concise with no unnecessary information.

Over the course of a paper the questions need to be independent of each other so that the answer to one question cannot become the key to solving another. Answers should all be of similar length, with no obviously wrong answers, and the position of the key in the list of distracters should vary randomly. Good distracters will be significantly different from the right answer and are statements that themselves contain true information, but which will not be relevant to the given question.

In the nMRCGP, approximately 80 per cent of question items will be on clinical medicine, 10 per cent on critical appraisal and evidence-based clinical practice and 10 per cent on health informatics and administrative issues. All questions will address important issues relating to UK general practice and will focus mainly on higher-order problem solving rather than just the simple recall of basic facts. RCGP policy for testing candidates' knowledge of research and of administration in primary care is that the current breadth of candidate knowledge required in these areas will remain unchanged from that in the outgoing MRCGP multiple-choice paper, as will the depth of knowledge.

Box 12.1 shows how candidates performed in the May 2007 diet of the multiple-choice paper.

BOX 12.1 Summary of outcomes in the May 2007 MRCGP multiple-choice paper

2159 candidates attempted the May 2007 multiple-choice question paper of the MRCGP. Their mean score was 145 out of 197 scored items (73.6 per cent), with the best candidate scoring 186 (94.4 per cent). The pass mark in this part of the MRCGP is regularly reviewed utilising internationally recognised statistical techniques for standard setting. The pass mark was set on this occasion at 131 (66.5 per cent) using a linear equating technique based on anchor items that have been used in previous test papers. This resulted in a pass rate of 79.2 per cent of those taking the paper.

On this occasion the merit mark was set at 159 out of the 197 scored items (80.7 per cent), and this was reached or exceeded by 24.7 per cent of candidates attempting the paper.

The mean scores by subject area were:

- research (including critical appraisal), 80.1 per cent
- administration and management, 64.0 per cent
- medicine, 73.3 per cent.

Reliability = 0.89

Standard error of measurement = 5.65 (2.87 per cent)

Poorly performing items
Three items performed poorly (i.e. they did not discriminate between good or poor candidates, or they were uniformly poorly answered). In one case this reflected recent changes in the recommended procedures for handling complaints in primary care NHS practice. These items were suppressed (i.e. they didn't contribute to the overall score), resulting in a total of 197 rather than 200 scored items.

Performance in key clinical areas

As is usual, candidates generally performed well in common and important areas such as the treatment of raised blood pressure, the investigation of respiratory conditions and the diagnosis of sexual problems. Areas of increasing clinical importance such as osteoporosis and hepatitis C were also answered well. Overall there were high scores in items testing research/administration.

Areas causing difficulty for candidates included child protection, paediatric asthma, anaphylaxis, palliative care and group B streptococcus in pregnancy.

Source: Dr Jo Richardson on behalf of all members of the RCGP MCP/AKT core group.

Questions are derived from accredited and referenced sources, including review articles and original papers in journals readily available to all general practitioners. These are primarily *Clinical Evidence, British Medical Journal, NICE Guidelines, British Journal of General Practice, Drug and Therapeutics Bulletin* or *Cochrane Reviews*.

Occasionally a question may use original material from published papers, and the item may take longer to complete. This variation in question time will have been taken into account in constructing the total paper.

The current edition of the *British National Formulary* is the reference source for therapeutics questions, including the general information on prescribing. Some questions may refer to the unlicensed but widely accepted use of specific drugs. Some of the questions relate to current best practice. They should be answered in relation to published evidence and not according to an individual's local arrangements.

BOX 12.2 Types of multiple-choice questions

There are two types of multiple-choice questions on the paper:

- extending matching questions (EMQ) in which a scenario has to be matched to an answer from a list of options. It may look as though there are several possible answers but the most likely answer should be selected from the option list

- single best answer (SBA) questions in which a statement or stem is followed by a variable number of items, only one of which is correct.

Below are some examples of AKT questions, taken from the RCGP website. These 22 questions should take about 20 minutes under exam conditions.

Extended matching questions

Theme: reduced vision

OPTION LIST

A ◊ Basilar migraine   F ◊ Occlusion of the central retinal vein
B ◊ Cerebral tumour   G ◊ Optic neuritis
C ◊ Cranial arteritis   H ◊ Retinal detachment
D ◊ Macular degeneration   I ◊ Tobacco optic neuropathy
E ◊ Occlusion of the central
    retinal artery

INSTRUCTION

For each patient with reduced vision, select the *single most likely* diagnosis. Each option may be used once, more than once, or not at all.

ITEMS

1 ◊ A 75-year-old man, who is a heavy smoker, with blood pressure of 170/105, complains of floaters in the right eye for many months and flashing lights in bright sunshine. He has now noticed a 'curtain' across the vision of his right eye.

2 ◊ A 70-year-old woman complains of shadows, which sometimes obscure her vision for a few minutes. She has felt unwell recently with loss of weight and face pain when chewing food.

3 ◊ A 45-year-old woman, who is a heavy smoker, with blood pressure of 170/110, complains of impaired vision in the left eye. She has difficulty discriminating colours and has noticed that her eye aches when looking to the side.

Theme: contraceptive advice

A ◊ 7 days of extra contraceptive precautions required.
B ◊ 14 days of extra contraceptive precautions required.
C ◊ Emergency contraception required.
D ◊ No extra precautions required.
E ◊ Omit pill-free week.

For each patient described below, select the *single most appropriate* statement of advice from the list above. Each option may be used once, more than once or not at all.

4 ◊ A 24-year-old woman is taking the combined contraceptive pill. She is on day 19 of the packet and rings to say that she forgot her pill yesterday morning and had intercourse last night. She has taken her pill this morning. Her last period was normal and she has taken all the other pills accurately.

5 ◊ A 36-year-old woman is taking the progesterone-only pill. She is on day 14 of the packet and rings to say that she forgot her pill yesterday and had intercourse last night. She has taken her pill this morning. Her last period was normal and she has taken all the other pills accurately.

6 ◊ A 28-year-old woman had her first baby eight weeks ago. She is not breast feeding and wishes to restart contraception straight away. She has not started menstruating yet has and receives her first dose of Depo-Provera that day.

7 ◊ A 26-year-old woman is taking the combined contraceptive pill. She forgot to start her new packet of pills three days ago and had intercourse last night. Her last period was normal and she had taken her previous pack of pills accurately.

8 ◊ A 24-year-old woman is taking the combined contraceptive pill. She is on day 19 of the packet and requires erythromycin for a skin infection as she is allergic to penicillin.

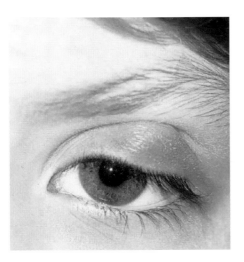

Single best answer

Theme: eye problems

9 ◊ A 42-year-old woman who has previously had treatment for cervical CIN 2 has had a lump affecting her left upper lid for three months (see picture). It is asymptomatic. What is the single most likely diagnosis in this patient? *Select one answer only*:

A ◊ entropion
B ◊ meibomian cyst
C ◊ metastatic deposit

D ◊ stye

E ◊ xanthelasma.

10 ◊ According to current evidence, in the management of croup in a 2-year-old child, which is the single most effective treatment to shorten the course of the condition? *Select one option only:*

A ◊ place the child in a steam-filled bathroom

B ◊ administer inhaled budesonide

C ◊ prescribe amoxicillin 125 mg t.d.s. for five days

D ◊ administer inhaled salbutamol

E ◊ prescribe paediatric cough suppressant containing codeine

F ◊ administer inhaled tribavirin.

11 ◊ Which one of the following plasma glucose levels (on two occasions) is diagnostic of diabetes mellitus? Select one option only:

A ◊ fasting plasma glucose > 5 mmol/L

B ◊ fasting plasma glucose > 6 mmol/L

C ◊ fasting plasma glucose > 7 mmol/L

D ◊ random plasma glucose > 10 mmol/L

E ◊ random plasma glucose > 9 mmol/L.

12 ◊ According to current evidence, which *one* of the following drugs produces the most significant reduction in menstrual flow for women with menorrhagia? *Select one option only:*

A ◊ diclofenac

B ◊ ethamsylate

C ◊ flurbiprofen

D ◊ mefenamic acid

E ◊ norethisterone

F ◊ tranexamic acid.

13 ◊ An 18-year-old patient presents with a two-day exacerbation of asthma following a worsening of hay fever. After using a salbutamol nebuliser her peak flow rate increases from 250 to 450 L/minute and she feels much better.

Which is the single most appropriate next management step? *Select one option only:*

A ◊ nebulised salbutamol as required

B ◊ no further treatment

C ◊ oral amoxicillin

D ◊ oral chlorphenamine

E ◊ oral prednisolone.

Table/algorithm completion is the format often found in guidelines to advise on management decisions. You are asked to select the correct answer to complete the table or diagram.

Theme: medical management of menorrhagia

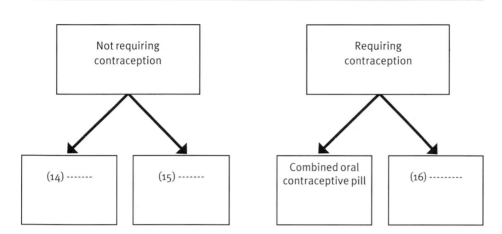

For each of the numbered gaps above, select *one* option from the list below to complete the algorithm, based on current evidence. *Select one option only*:

A ◊ copper intrauterine device
B ◊ cyclical medroxyprogesterone acetate
C ◊ cyclical norethisterone
D ◊ inert intrauterine device
E ◊ levonorgestrel-releasing intrauterine system
F ◊ mefenamic acid
G ◊ nonoxinol '9'
H ◊ tibolone
I ◊ tranexamic acid.

Theme: NHS breast-screening referral guidelines

For each numbered question, select the *correct* option to complete the algorithm from the list below. Each answer may be used once, more than once or not at all (the diagram for this question follows):

A ◊ age 25
B ◊ age 35
C ◊ age 45
D ◊ age 55
E ◊ discrete lump

F ◊ dominant asymmetrical nodularity
G ◊ symmetrical nodularity
H ◊ refer
I ◊ review
J ◊ reassure.

132

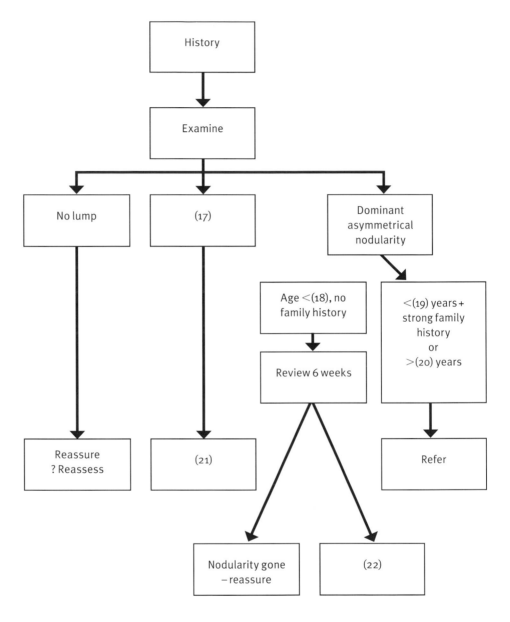

So we can see that the AKT looks at that baseline knowledge essential for safe practice as well as the ability to apply that knowledge. The best way to prepare for the AKT exam is certainly to be well read in the main general practice reference literature and up to date with current best practice. In addition it will be important to frequently engage in discussions with doctors and others to develop and apply that knowledge to real-life situations.

Trainees, not unnaturally, have a great sense of urgency towards identifying the 'right answers', especially at exam preparation time. Trainers can best help trainees develop into self-directed learners and ultimately independent practitioners by the way in which they respond to this and the type of teaching and learning opportunities they guide their trainees towards. With experience it becomes clear that there is often not one 'right answer' when helping patients make choices about their health. So learning that reinforces this variation will be the best preparation for the future, rather than rote learning for written exams. Case-based discussions (CbDs) and the consultation observation tool (COT) of Workplace-Based Assessment (WPBA) will be ways by which trainers and clinical supervisors can guide trainees towards acquiring important information and ways of applying that knowledge.

The AKT is however the response to the need to ensure trainees have a safe level of applied knowledge. In preparation, practice with multiple-choice questions can be excellent as a needs assessment tool to identify areas for further study. The RCGP has developed one such tool in the PEP eKit. This is an online interactive test aimed at helping doctors to identify strengths, weaknesses and specific educational needs. The topics covered are ophthalmology, ENT, dermatology, general medicine, psychiatry, paediatrics, and obstetrics and gynaecology. As with all aspects of GP training the art is finding the balance between different types of learning activity.

For the last five diets of the MRCGP multiple-choice paper, the College has given general feedback on the standard of candidates' performance on the website. This will continue under the AKT, and will further help trainers and educationalists support GPStRs.

Multi-source feedback

David Bruce and Joan Sargeant

While scientific advances in medicine continue to offer more possibilities for high-tech and complex interventions, the effectiveness of our practice remains embedded in our relationships with patients and colleagues. Our goal of person-centred care requires understanding of individuals and their unique context, respect, empathy and involvement. It also requires working collaboratively with clinicians and non-clinicians to provide that care. As a result, there is considerable interest in measurements that give information on these humanistic and collaborative components of medical performance in addition to clinical capability. Multi-source feedback (MSF) is one such assessment format.

MSF, also known as 360° evaluation, was developed in the private sector as successful businesses acknowledged the need to adapt and respond to the environments in which they operated.[1] To encourage this adaptation, they developed a system of providing feedback on performance and behaviours to individual managers from work colleagues, i.e. their supervisors, peers and staff, and from customers as appropriate. MSF uses questionnaires completed by those working closely with individuals being assessed to collect and compile data about their performance).[2]

Within the context of GP training in the UK, it can be defined as:

A specific instrument designed to gather information on clinical capability and professional behaviours of the learner. Observers may include medical, nursing and allied health professional staff, and within the general practice setting, non clinical staff such as reception staff and practice managers. Feedback is provided in aggregate form and is used to provide formative assessment and help identify learners in difficulty.

Administrative details about the MSF are available on the RCGP website at www.rcgp.org.uk/the_gp_journey/nmrcgp/wpba_tools/msf.aspx.

This chapter will cover three main areas: the background and research evidence for use of MSF for performance assessment and feedback, the two-question MSF tool used in Workplace-Based Assessment (WPBA), and a framework for facilitating feedback generated by the MSF tool. We will also include a guidance section for non-clinical raters.

Background and evidence for use of MSF

The intent of MSF as an assessment approach is formative and developmental, to provide guidance for continued learning and practice improvement. To this end, basic assumptions about MSF include the following:

1 ◊ the rigour of the MSF tool is ensured through reliability and validity testing
2 ◊ reviewing the compiled feedback from colleagues and co-workers will raise participants' awareness of their performance and how others see them
3 ◊ feedback indicating a need for practice change will lead to that change.

We will briefly explore each of these assumptions in light of the literature. Regarding the rigour of MSF tools, a variety of tools has been developed and psychometrically tested in the UK and North America, primarily used for assessing and providing feedback to registrars/residents and practising doctors. Such testing has determined the validity of individual tools, the factors or domains included in each, and their reliability and generalisability, the latter identifying the number of items and raters required for a rigorous assessment.

Regarding the influence of MSF upon increasing participants' awareness of their performance and subsequent practice improvement, research findings are mixed and point to the need for further work. Drawing upon research in organisational psychology, participants focusing upon positive, not negative, aspects of feedback were more likely to accept it and improve.[3] Alternatively, negative feedback can be perceived as inaccurate and lead to distress, demoralisation and demotivation instead of motivation for change. A meta-analysis of appraisal studies of managers demonstrated that the performance of one third actually declined for these reasons.[4]

Within medicine, results of MSF research are similar. Notably, studies show that MSF can result in positive changes by the majority of participants and these changes are primarily in communication and patient information.[5,6] However, not all receiving negative feedback accepted it or changed, as they did not see it as consistent with self-perceptions and some reacted with distress that could be strong and longstanding.[7] In another study, poor performers rated themselves higher than their colleagues did, suggesting that those most likely to receive negative feedback may be the least likely to benefit from it.[8]

Factors influencing the acceptance and use of MSF

A number of factors have been found in industry to influence the use of MSF, including, among others, characteristics of the feedback, the recipient's initial reactions, personality (especially degree of self-monitoring), beliefs about change, perceived need for change, goal setting.[9] Other research points to the need for the assessment to be fair, which is often as much about how the assessment is administered rather than the outcomes, i.e. procedural *vs* distributive

justice.[10] This is substantiated by medical research, which found that perceptions of MSF credibility and fairness highly influenced its acceptance and use,
as did its specificity. Specific, credible feedback is more readily used.[6] Finally,
the role of the trainer is paramount especially if feedback is perceived to be
negative and skills in facilitation are required. Indeed it is suggested that relationship between the trainee and trainer may be the main agent of change rather
than the feedback itself.[1]

The two-question MSF

Development

The development of the two-question MSF has drawn on previous work in
MSF. It can be viewed on the RCGP website. Medical MSF tools aim to rate
a doctor's performance over a variety of domains. For each MSF tool the individual items are usually highly correlated and, using the statistical technique
factor analysis, have been shown in some studies to collapse down to two main
dimensions, clinical and cognitive ability and humanistic qualities.[11,12] This
would seem to fit with day-to-day experience; if asked by a relative of friend for
an opinion on a doctor, the main thoughts when answering are 'What are they
like clinically?' and 'What are they like as an individual?' With this in mind the
two-question MSF sets out to rate clinical ability and professional behaviour.

Measurement research indicates that, when using a smaller number of items
(two questions), increasing the number of observations can provide adequate
reliability.[13] The two-question MSF is therefore used on two occasions, a minimum of two months apart. This allows for the trainees' progress as well as performance to be tracked. The reliability of an assessment is the degree to which
it is able to differentiate between candidates, and is a requirement for a fair and
valid assessment. Pilot work in nine UK deaneries has demonstrated this MSF
has high reliability with five clinical and five non-clinical raters on two occasions.[14] These results give credibility to the MSF tool and allow confidence in
the feedback results.

Given that delivery of primary care is a whole-team venture it is important
to include non-clinical staff as raters. Although it is inappropriate to ask non-
clinicians to rate trainees' clinical ability, it is realistic to believe that professional
behaviour – including aspects such as respect for individuals and the ability
to work in a team – can indeed be accurately rated by non-clinical GP staff. In
fact, research supports this assumption. It is also postulated that in some cases
behaviours may differ towards non-clinical staff than to the GP trainer and
partners, so inclusion of the non-clinical staff in the MSF adds an important
dimension. Indeed the high reliability of the MSF using only non-clinical staff
backs this idea.[14]

However, as noted in the previous section, for MSF to work feedback must also be specific.[6] Having only two items reduces specificity and, to counteract this, free-text boxes have been added in which raters provide specific comments about performance. For each of the two questions, in addition to the numerical rating, there are two obligatory free-text boxes:

- *highlights in performance (areas to be commended)*
- *suggested areas for development in performance.*

138

Free text is a crucial part of the two-question MSF as it is the source of more specific feedback. It is therefore imperative that trainers encourage all those taking part as raters in the trainee's MSF to include comments in the free-text boxes. The more specific the information, the more value the feedback will be to the trainee. Experience from the pilot indicated that both clinical and non-clinical raters were happy to provide free-text comments.

Through completion of the MSF by clinical and non-clinical staff, and completion of the patient satisfaction questionnaire (PSQ) (described in detail in Chapter 14) by patients, the trainee should receive comprehensive feedback about both clinical and humanistic/professional clinical performance.

When to use the MSF

ST1

The two-question MSF is used at month 4 and 6 in ST1. As previously explained, two iterations are required for reliability. It is likely, at least for the first year or so of the new GP specialist training, that those in ST1 will be training in a hospital environment. For hospital posts only, the MSF will be rated by five clinical staff on the two occasions. When the doctor is working in the training practice five clinical and five non-clinical staff will be raters, thereby involving the wider primary healthcare team.

ST3

As the final year of GP specialist training will be spent in general practice, the two-question MSF will be used at months 28–30 and then 2–4 months later. Five clinicians and five non-clinicians will be raters.

Some important notes are that:

- in both years the same or different raters can be used on each occasion
- clinician raters answer both questions (professional behaviour, clinical ability)
- non-clinician raters answer only question (professional behaviour).

How to use the MSF

The trainee selects colleagues and invites them to participate as raters in their MSF. He or she provides the participants with an instruction letter on the MSF available from the RCGP website (www.rcgp.org.uk/the_gp_journey/nmrcgp/wpba_tools/msf.aspx).

Raters log into the RCGP web page and enter the trainee's name and GMC number, then completing the e-form. The process of inviting raters and having them complete the form should take no longer than two weeks.

BOX 13.1 **Tips for educational supervisors and trainers**

The quality of feedback provided is determined by raters' free-text comments. You need to encourage all to write comments and to be as specific as possible.

Reassure all staff that the MSF is completely anonymous and comments cannot be traced to any individual.

As trainer you need to be aware which colleagues have been asked to participate by your trainee.

If you feel that those chosen are not fully representative of your practice then this should be discussed with your trainee.

You are required to check that those asked did indeed complete the MSF form.

The results of the MSF are initially accessed by the trainer before being released to the GPStR. This screening allows planning of the feedback interview, with appropriate timescale to allow the trainee to reflect on the results.

The feedback cannot be altered or censored.

Non-clinical raters can potentially find the invitation to pass comment on GPStRs challenging. The power differential between doctors and employees such as receptionists or ward staff can mean that their comments are either too non-specific or confined to observations about superficial issues. One way to ensure comments are robust and useful will be linked to the development of a supportive learning environment, and will depend on the practice or hospital culture about the openness of professional relationships. An effective educational supervisor will be paying attention to those aspects of the environment that can lead to increased honesty and utility of the feedback from non-clinical raters. You may also wish to consider giving general feedback to raters about the value of their contributions.

Providing feedback on the MSF data

To achieve our goal of person-centred care it is important that the views of patients and colleagues form a part of a global assessment of performance and progress of doctors in training. The following are concerns highlighted in the literature regarding the provision and acceptance of feedback:

- positive evaluations are perceived to be more accurate than negative ones
- those focusing on the positive aspects are most likely to improve
- being ranked as below the average results in loss of positive feelings
- individuals may not see the need to change when unfavorable feedback is at odds with their own self-perceptions
- those who rate themselves higher or lower than others may have less insight
- negative rankings often do not increase self-awareness
- negative rankings can result in anger and de-motivation.

In light of these concerns, we need to consider how it is possible to best facilitate the trainee receiving, accepting and using their MSF evaluation. For this we draw upon psychological change and therapeutic counselling constructs, which suggest using a coaching model.[1]

A coaching model seems to work best in resolving the differences between self-perceptions and the views of others, and using them as a driver for change, facilitating the assimilation of feedback and helping to plan for change.

Based on current evidence we propose a three-part feedback framework for use with the MSF. This model is also suitable for use in facilitation of feedback from the PSQ.

The feedback framework

The framework consists of the following:

1 ◊ setting the scene
2 ◊ preparation and planning
3 ◊ feedback facilitation – the ECO model.

1 □ Setting the scene

This starts right at the beginning of training. When agreeing on the educational contract with the trainee, the MSF tool should be explained and discussed. This should include how and when it will be used and explore the trainee's attitudes towards the tool and its use. The purpose of the tool (to identify areas for development), the credibility of the tool (the research evidence, use of non-clinical colleagues, free-text responses) and the normal sensitivity that one feels about comments regarding one's contribution and ability are key discussion areas. This touches upon aspects of the psychological contract with the trainee – the often unsaid assumptions of what is required from the trainee by the practice and what the trainee requires in return.

2 □ *Preparation and planning*

BY THE TRAINER

- Ensure feedback provided is constructive, i.e. is specific, is timely, describes and does not judge, and is given with genuineness and empathy.
- The nature of the feedback needs to be considered. Is it positive, negative or a mix?
- Look at the specific comments and consider in light of these what challenges may arise.
- Consider how much time for reflection on the results should be given to the trainee before your feedback meeting. Research shows that having some time to reflect on one's own, especially if feedback is negative, enhances both emotional and cognitive assimilation of the feedback.

BY THE TRAINEE

- The trainee needs to review and consider the feedback.
- The trainee should reflect upon 'How does this differ my self-evaluation?' What are the specific comments and what are the opportunities for improvements?

3 □ *Feedback facilitation – the ECO model*

This interview is the key part in the process if a positive outcome and change is to result. A simple three-part model, E (emotional response), C (content of feedback) and O (outcomes), can be visually represented as traffic lights — a stop, get ready and go moment on the trainee's learning journey (see Figure 13.2 on p. 142). For some this will be an exacting session needing all the trainer's skills, so an *aide-mémoire* may be of help. Questions to help at each stage are contained in the MEMO box, which is expanded in Box 13.3 (see p. 143).

E ◊ EMOTIONAL RESPONSE (goal: emotional readiness to move on)

Here the task is to encourage the trainee to reflect on his or her emotions on receiving the MSF responses. Is this what the trainee expected, i.e. is it consistent with his or her own self-assessment of his or her performance? The trainer should probe, clarify and challenge as appropriate. In the case of negative feedback, it is important to 'allow' distress and not to jump to the rescue. The outcome of this stage is that the trainee is at a stage of emotional readiness to move ahead and consider the content of the feedback. Closure may not be possible at this time, but the trainee should feel that his or her distress is understood and he or she feels supported. Awareness-raising questions provided in the MEMO box are helpful.

FIGURE 13.2 **The ECO model**

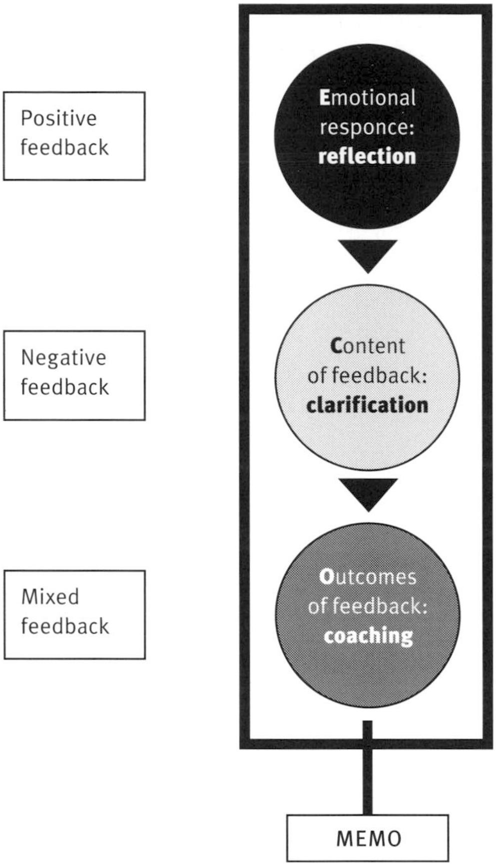

Positive feedback

Negative feedback

Mixed feedback

Emotional responce: **reflection**

Content of feedback: **clarification**

Outcomes of feedback: **coaching**

MEMO

C ◊ CLARIFYING CONTENT (goal: clarity in understanding feedback content)
Here trainees are encouraged to reflect on the feedback and their interpretation of the specific comments, and to describe in their own words the feedback messages in terms of their own specific performance. The trainer's role should again be to explore, clarify and challenge if appropriate. Again the MEMO box questions are helpful.

O ◊ OUTCOMES (goal: outcomes and plan agreed)
At this stage engage the trainee in identifying leaning needs and goals for improvement of performance based upon the specific feedback. It is important to identify barriers to changes and develop a positive action plan, with follow-up review timescale agreed (see MEMO box questions).

Broadly the three groups of feedback recipients (positive, negative and mix) will have different challenges. Whilst it is likely that those receiving positive feedback will find the feedback credible and accurate, this may not be the case for those receiving negative feedback. Remember for the mixed group that most doctors rate themselves as above the average, so even mixed or average feedback may be perceived as mostly negative. For each grouping therefore, more time may be required at the particular stages of the ECO model. All groups should be able to develop a plan for improvement.

143

BOX 13.3 **The MEMO box – helpful questions and phrases for each step**

Step 1 ◊ emotional response – reflection
- ☐ 'It sounds like this feedback was a surprise for you. Can you tell me more about that?'
- ☐ 'Most people find it tough when they first receive feedback that differs from their own perceptions.'
- ☐ 'Because it's a surprise, it often takes a little while to adjust to it.'
- ☐ 'We all think we're doing our best and it's hard when others give us a different view.'
- ☐ 'Are there specific aspects of it that are difficult for you? Tell me about them.'
- ☐ 'Can you reflect back and think why you might have received this score?'
- ☐ 'Are there some bits of your feedback that you can perhaps accept and start to work on?'

Step 2 ◊ content of feedback – clarification
- ☐ 'Is there any of this feedback that you're unclear about? Any items that don't make sense to you?'
- ☐ 'Tell me in your own words how it relates to your practice.'
- ☐ 'Can you give examples of your performance that might relate to this item/section that might have resulted in this score or comment?'

Step 3 ◊ outcomes of feedback – coaching an action plan
- ☐ 'Does any of this feedback suggest a way you might wish to improve your performance/ what you're doing in a particular area?'
- ☐ 'Most of us can improve on our performance in one area or another. Does this feedback suggest any specific opportunities for you?'
- ☐ 'How might you go about making that improvement?'
- ☐ 'Do you need any resources or additional learning to do that? Are they accessible to you?'
- ☐ 'What's a reasonable timeline for making the change?'
- ☐ 'How will you know you've succeeded? What will be the indicator/s of success?'

Note: for steps 2 and 3 especially, focusing upon specific feedback, not generalities, is most helpful.

REFERENCES

1. Goodstone MS, Diamante T. Organizational use of therapeutic change: strengthening multisource feedback systems through interdisciplinary coaching *Consulting Psychology Journal: practice and research* 1998; 50(3): 152–63.

2. Bracken DW, Timmreck CW, Church AH. *The Handbook of Multi Source Feedback: the comprehensive resource for designing and implementing MSF processes* San Francisco: Jossey-Bass, 2001.

3. McFarland C, Miller DT. The framing of relative performance feedback: seeing the glass half empty or half full *Journal of Personality and Social Psychology* 1994; 66: 1061–73.

4. Kluger AN, DeNisi A. The effects of feedback interventions on performance: a historical review, a meta-analysis, and a preliminary feedback intervention theory *Psychological Bulletin* 1996; 119(2): 254–84.

5. Lockyer J. Multisource feedback in the assessment of physician competencies *Journal of Continuing Education in the Health Professions* 2003; 23: 4–12.

6. Sargeant J, Mann K, Sinclair D, *et al*. Challenges in multi-source feedback: intended and unintended outcomes *Medical Education* 2007; 41(6): 583–91.

7. Sargeant J, Mann K, Sinclair D, *et al*. Understanding the influence of emotions and reflection upon multi-source feedback acceptance and use *Advances in Health Science Education* 2006; 10.1007/s10459-006-9039-x.

8. Violato C, Lockyer J. Self and peer assessment of paediatricians, psychiatrists and medicine specialists: implications for self directed learning *Advances in Health Science Education* 2006; 11: 235–44.

9. Smither JW, London M, Reilly RR. Does performance improve following multisource feedback? A theoretical model, meta-analysis and review of empirical findings *Personnel Psychology* 2005; 58: 33–66.

10. van den Boss K, Vermunt R, Wilke AM. Procedural and distributive justice: what is fair depends more on what comes first than on what comes next *Journal of Personality and Social Psychology* 1997; 72(1): 95–104.

11. Ramsay P, Wenrich MD, Carline JD, *et al*. Use of peer ratings to evaluate physician performance *Journal of the American Medical Association* 1993; 269(13): 1655–60.

12. Dannefer EF, Henson CH, Bierer SB, *et al*. Peer assessment of professional competence *Medical Education* 2005; 39: 713–22.

13. Williams RG, Verhulst S, Colliver JA, *et al*. Assessing the reliability of resident performance appraisals: more items or more observations? *Surgery* 2005; 137: 141–7.

14. Murphy DJ, Bruce DA, Eva K. *Workplace Based Assessment for nMRCGP: external tools pilot report 2005–2006*, www.dundee.ac.uk/gptraining/Workplace%20Asst/Workplace%20Asst%20Downloads.htm [accessed December 2007].

144

14 Patient satisfaction questionnaire

Amar Rughani

The Postgraduate Medical Education and Training Board (PMETB) has been a great driver for change in medical assessments and one of the most important of its exhortations is principle five, which states that *'Assessments must provide relevant feedback'*. This principle reflects the fact that assessment brings learners face to face with their performance and that this creates a powerful incentive for improvement *provided* that relevant feedback can be given and, just as importantly, given in the appropriate way.

Feedback is therefore the link between assessment and ongoing learning. In this chapter, we will look at the technique of giving feedback in relation to the patient satisfaction questionnaire (PSQ).

What is the PSQ?

The Consultation and Relational Empathy (CARE) measure was developed by Dr Stewart Mercer and colleagues as part of a Health Services Research Fellowship funded by the Chief Scientist Office of the Scottish Executive (2000–2003). It is based on a validated tool that probes the patient's perception of the doctor's relational empathy within the consultation.[1]

The questionnaire is a compulsory part of Workplace-Based Assessment (WPBA) and details of how it is administered can be found on the RCGP website, www.rcgp.org.uk/the_gp_journey/nmrcgp/wpba_tools/psq.aspx.

TIP

Take a minute to look up the questions in the PSQ on the website, before reading further.

How can the PSQ be interpreted?

The results on which the educator gives feedback are presented as the mean, median and range for each question. These three figures can be helpful in the following ways:

Mean

This indicates the average score.

Median

This indicates the middle score when the scores are presented in numerical order. Sometimes the median can be more helpful than the mean in trying to work out what the 'average' is, for example when the average score might be skewed because one or more results are very different from the majority.

Range

This is represented by the standard deviation (SD). If the standard deviation is low, this suggests that most of the scores are quite close to each other. If the SD is high, there is a much greater spread. Another way of putting this is that when the SD is low, most patients are in agreement with each other, whereas when the SD is high, there is a relative lack of consensus. In the latter situation, we can't be as certain that the average score as represented by the mean is a true reflection of the doctor's performance.

When looking at the data, it is probably better to start with the big picture and then zoom in to consider the detail. Here is a possible sequence of events:

- what can we learn from the mean, median and standard deviation? As we have described, we can establish whether the mean and median marks on which we decide strengths/weaknesses are a fair reflection of the learner's performance. If the standard deviation is high, there may be too large a spread to be certain although, in most cases, this would not be the case
- what is the overall rating? Question 11 provides a global impression of the doctor's performance and this sets the scene for what follows. For example, even if areas of weakness are identified, if the doctor's performance is rated overall as being 'very good' then the doctor deserves to feel pleased. The converse is also true
- what are the areas of strength and weakness? PSQ provides evidence of ability in four competence areas of WPBA, as shown in Table 14.1.

Q		Communication and consultation skills	Practising holistically	Managing medical complexity and promoting health	Maintaining an ethical approach to practice
1	Feel at ease	X			X
2	Tell 'your' story	X			
3	Really listening	X			X
4	Interested in whole person		X		
5	Understanding your concerns	X			X
6	Showing care				X
7	Being positive			X	
8	Explaining clearly	X			
9	Helping you take control			X	
10	Making a plan together	X			

TABLE 14.1 **The competence areas addressed by the PSQ**

As we can see, two of these areas dominate and, although they overlap, we may be able to analyse how the learner is performing in each of them separately. This exercise is worth doing because it can help us to be more focused in our feedback and help the learner to be more specific in developing his or her learning plan.

- How does this information fit with what is already known? The learner is more likely to take notice of the feedback if it confirms what is already known about him or her. If it seems to be at odds, then further action may need to be taken such as looking at patient feedback again, checking communication skills through COT and looking at feedback from colleagues through MSF. These will help the educator and learner decide whether a significant learning need exists.
- What are the learning needs and how good is the learner's insight? It is important to note that a score of 4 on any question is equivalent to 'good' and is therefore unlikely to suggest that a significant learning need is present.

Check with the learner to see whether the score is roughly in line with his or her own self-assessment. This helps to gauge the learner's insight and establish whether the learner has good judgement or whether he or she has more confidence or less confidence in his or her ability than might be appropriate.

What factors influence the impact of feedback?

The purpose of giving feedback is to encourage learners to change and improve. Therefore it is helpful to know what factors influence the impact that feedback might have. Through understanding this, we can tailor our feedback to achieve its intended purpose.

Learners are more likely to change behaviour if feedback anticipates learners' concerns, some of which may be unspoken. This may have an influence on the impact of feedback.

If we find that giving feedback on performance is not going well, it is worth exploring any underlying concerns, particularly the unspoken ones.

- Is the group who gave the feedback credible to the GP specialty registrar (GPStR)? Although receiving feedback from patients is compulsory, we should not assume that learners accept that patients are credible reviewers. It may seem obvious that patients can comment upon communication and empathy, but it may be worth asking learners about their views, particularly if they have not been trained in the UK, have been brought up in another culture or do not appear at ease with the concept.
- Is the feedback specific enough? To be effective, feedback should be specific enough for learners to formulate SMART learning objectives (see also Chapter 4). Feedback should focus on facts and on behaviours, rather than on personality.
- The GPStR may not feel the need to change. Objectively, a need may be inferred from the scores and from comparison between the scores and what the learner already knows about his or her performance from other sources.[2] However, whether the learner feels *committed* to change depends upon motivational forces. We will explore these below.
- Is feedback being given in an appropriate way? If feedback is given poorly, which sadly has often been the case in medicine, it can be destructive (see Chapter 4).[3,4]
- Learners respond well to positive advice and (being human) have a tendency to ignore negative comments! Therefore, it can be more effective to assign 'commendation flags' to good scores and 'information flags' to poor ones.
- Have goals been set? Feedback alone is not enough. For learners to change, they need to set their own goals to which they have a sense of commitment.[5]
- Is there follow-up? The literature shows that supporting the learner beyond the initial discussion can greatly help to increase performance.[6] Educators can do this by encouraging the development of goals, supporting progress and celebrating achievement.

Motivating the learner

What is the purpose of giving feedback? There is a danger that we might attend to the process without asking this fundamental question. Feedback may help learners to see where they need to learn, but knowing what to do and wanting to do it are two separate, although related, items. The maximum gain occurs when both are addressed. Therefore, as well as using feedback skills to interpret PSQ, educators can use similar skills to address the learner's motivation for improvement.

149

Let's use an analogy. Figure 14.1 shows our learner who, with the help of his educator, is choosing to swim rather than sink.

FIGURE 14.1 **Factors affecting a swimmer's progress**

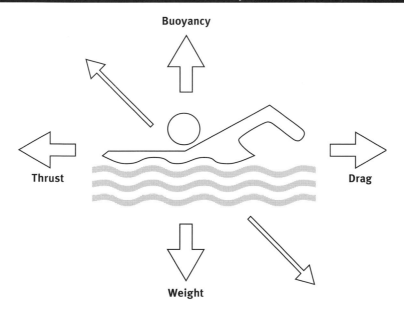

Motivation, or the ability to swim in our analogy, is not simply one force with one direction, but is the outcome of a number of influences. Understanding this is useful because it gives us a number of ways, rather than simply one way, of helping the learner move in a positive direction. We might think of motivation as being helped by:

1 ◊ THE THRUST ◊ or the power that learners have to propel themselves forward. The main source of thrust is often a commitment to a specific goal. In the context of PSQ, this might be a perceived need to change based on the feedback. If the need is not apparent, we might probe what the doctor understands or feels about the common drivers of need such as pressure of the exam, peer pressure or a desire to improve patient care

2 ◊ BUOYANCY ◊ which can help with forward motion. This could be a belief in success. Often, this buoyancy provides the lift that initiates movement in a positive direction. As educators, we can influence buoyancy by helping learners to appreciate their positive attributes and previous successes. We can increase their confidence and point out the positive factors that might aid success, such as the availability of guidance or resources.

Motivation might be hindered by:

1 ◊ WEIGHT ◊ or the baggage that the learner carries, such as a lack of confidence or a previous negative experience. Educators can help by probing whether such hindrances exist and by discussing these or signposting other forms of help that might be available

2 ◊ DRAG ◊ which comes from factors that actively hold the learner back. In PSQ, 'drag' may be caused by external factors such as a lack of opportunity to learn, for example courses or study leave. More importantly, drag may come from internal factors that may or may not be perceived by the learner, such as lack of understanding of communication skills or lack of insight into one's own unhelpful attitudes. Again, educators can be invaluable in helping learners to see that drag is an issue with everyone and in helping learners to identify their own sources.

Figure 14.1 shows how motivation is the resultant of two opposing forces represented by the arrows. Very often, educators are good at attending to goals but we are less good at recognising goals, i.e. thrust. By augmenting the force of the top-left arrow and simultaneously reducing the negative effect of the bottom-right arrow, learners can be helped to propel themselves with remarkable power, with benefit of themselves and patient care alike.

This chapter summarises the key role of the trainer in giving feedback. The data from the PSQ is important to help the GPStR develop but we can see that inexpertly handled feedback might risk losing this opportunity.

REFERENCES

1. Mercer S, Maxwell M, Heaney D, *et al*. The consultation and relational empathy (CARE) measure: development and preliminary validation and reliability of an empathy-based consultation process measure *Family Practice* 2004; 21(6): 699–705.

2. Johnson JW, Ferstl KL. The effects of interrater and self–other agreement on performance improvement following upward feedback *Personnel Psychology* 1999; 52: 271–303.

3. Hewson MG, Little ML. Giving feedback in medical education: verification of recommended techniques *Journal of General Internal Medicine* 1998; 13(2): 111–16.

4. Holmboe ES, Yepes M, Williams F, *et al*. Feedback and the mini clinical evaluation exercise *Journal of General Internal Medicine* 2004; 19: 558–61.

5. Locke EA, Latham GP. *A Theory of Goal Setting and Task Performance* Englewood Cliffs, NJ: Prentice Hall, 1990.

6. Walker AG, Smither JW. A five-year study of upward feedback: what managers do with their results matters *Personnel Psychology* 1999; 52: 393–423.

15 Planning learning in the new curriculum

Mike Deighan and Kay Mohanna

The most important change with the new curriculum is that responsibility for planning education now lies explicitly with the learner and not with the teacher. This is not to say that the clinical or educational supervisors have no role at all. They are still responsible for ensuring that learning takes place, but rather than planning content the trainer should focus on the structure and processes of learning. In short they must create a self-directed learner. This is not likely to be an easy task. Many learners are used to having their education packaged for them and will take some time to adjust to the notion of planning their own education. In addition, not all educators are comfortable with the concept of letting learners plan and direct their own learning, fearing that learners will only attend to aspects that interest them, or that they find easy, and that important areas will be left untouched.

In this chapter we will discuss planning of learning. We will look at how a GPStR can be encouraged to take, and make the most of, learning opportunities both 'on the job' and 'off the job', seeking and optimising the use of available resources. We will consider just in time learning, the place of web-based and blending learning, and small-group learning (learning sets).

Learner-centred planning

Four linked developments in the new curriculum are important in planning the professional development of trainees:

1. ◊ the fact that the new curriculum is outcomes based
2. ◊ the use of Personal Development Plans (PDPs)
3. ◊ the use of formative assessment in the workplace
4. ◊ provision of choice in learning.

Outcomes-based curriculum

One of the strengths of outcomes-based curricula is that they clearly set out for learners what they have to do to achieve success. This allows learners to orientate themselves, to identify their learning needs and to create plans of how to achieve their goals. They can also self-monitor their progress against the criteria.

However, in learning the art of general practice, outcomes-based education has limitations. Stenhouse[1] warns of two dangers when we oversimplify curricula into objectives. First, we can distort the content of our teaching to fit the objectives, destroying the unity of the whole by breaking chunks that fit with objectives. Second, we risk sending a message to the learner that once they have achieved the written curriculum outcomes they have mastered the art of general practice. It is well to remember that mastering the art amounts to more than achieving the learning objectives set down in the curriculum.

In particular for those GPStRs in ST1 and ST2, the personal development that occurs in hospital placements is not confined to picking up those aspects of that specialty that will be useful in practice. It also includes acquisition of generic competences.

Personal Development Plans

Planning is part of the experiential learning cycle of Kolb: testing learning in new situations and planning to repeat actions modified in the light of experience (see Figure 15.1).[2]

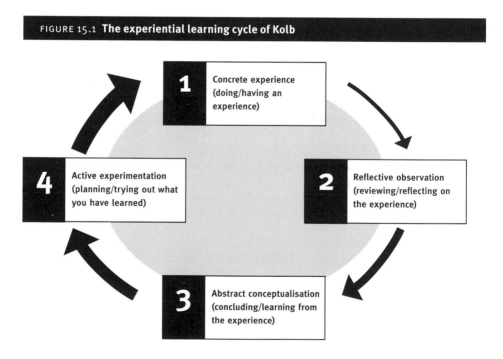

FIGURE 15.1 The experiential learning cycle of Kolb

Source: text and concept by Clara Davies/tutorial design by Tony Lowe. Copyright University of Leeds.

PDPs are predicated on the experiential model of learning, and encourage learners to plan future learning by reflecting on experience. They are part of the current educational strategy for training and, as part of his or her Workplace-Based Assessment (WPBA), each trainee has to produce an annual PDP.

Honey and Mumford[3] suggest that some people have learning styles preferences for part of the cycle whilst disliking or even avoiding other parts. For example, some doctors like to try new experiences and are averse to reflection, whereas others prefer to think and reflect, and may be reticent to try new ways of doing things.

It is important to recognise that planning education does not appeal to all trainees, some preferring to make the most of incidental learning. Not every learner will want to produce a PDP or find it an experience he or she values. In a well-argued article that questions the whole strategy of PDPs, Jennings[4] writes about doctors who do not enjoy planned learning (yet are still good adult learners), and doctors who like producing learning plans and have well-constructed portfolios (but rarely action their plans). He writes:

the paradox of the PDP is that it is potentially a useful learning tool for those to whom it holds least appeal but who need a structured approach – holist activist/pragmatists, who tend to include on it tasks they have already completed; it is probably of no use to those analyst/theorist-reflectors who have their own more detailed portfolio anyway, but quite enjoy filling in the PDP.

He suggests that to be useful, a PDP should be 'short term, tailored to the individual and incorporate strategic challenges'.

Box 15.1 summarises the role of the PDP in the GPStRs' training.

BOX 15.1 The trainee's PDP

A PDP is not a rigid plan of the education for that year; it is a document that reflects the current view on the direction of travel and may be modified in the light of developments during the year. It is not the sum total of the education for the year, but a series of milestones that are part of his or her journey towards independent practice as a general practitioner.

Formative assessment and assessment in the national tests (Applied Knowledge Test and Clinical Skills Assessment)

The timing of the Applied Knowledge Test (AKT) and Clinical Skills Assessment (CSA) is likely to be the first topic on the agenda at the annual appraisal and each will make their way into the PDP.

Planning for the AKT

It is not the trainer's role to provide teaching in factual knowledge for the GPStR. Like all other doctors, GP trainees need to develop their own study skills for keeping their knowledge up to date. Trainers and educational supervisors have a minor role in supervising the progress of the GPStR in preparing for the AKT, identifying suitable books and online resources, setting aside time for personal study or computer-based learning and monitoring the progress of their trainee towards self-directedness.

Planning for the CSA

The trainer has a much more important role in preparing the trainee for the CSA. First, it is crucial that the learner sees the connection between the CSA and WPBA. The best preparation for the CSA is for trainees to develop excellent communication skills and develop a clear understanding of what is happening during their consultations. The consultation observation tool (COT) is the mechanism for developing communication skills. The case-based discussion (CbD) is where they come to understand the complexities of general practice by examining their diagnostic and management decision making, and learn from their experiences.

So, to learn from their experience of consulting, trainees should plan to see as many patients as possible, and do lots of COTs and CbDs. As with all experiential learning, it is more efficient to use all parts of the Kolb cycle. To ensure development and quality learning, the trainer should:

1 ◊ encourage self-assessment by the learner
2 ◊ provide high-quality feedback (formative assessment)
3 ◊ encourage learners to use that feedback in their subsequent consultation (this is done by focusing on a particular theme over a series of COTs or CbDs).

This feedback is crucial in driving learning forward. Box 15.2 summarises how this can be achieved.

Assessment for learning

We cannot plan for learning until we know the trainee's needs, but how are these learning needs established? We know there is overwhelming evidence that doctors are incapable of assessing their learning needs accurately.[4] Confidence rating scales are of little use; to build an accurate picture, we need to look at what GPStRs can do, and not what they think they can do. Needs are best discovered by watching trainees consulting and listening to their ideas on their cases. A good way to achieve this is by formative use of COT and CbD. (These

BOX 15.2 **Using COT and CbD in a formative way in the workplace**

- Formative assessment is when subsequent learning changes as a result of the assessment.

- COTs and CbDs are a way of talking to trainees about what they need to learn.

- Early in the first GP attachment, use COTs and CbDs frequently and focus on feedback rather than on grading.

- There will be a tendency for GPStRs to look at their grades and not at their feedback. They need to be reminded that WPBA is the documentation of the progression over time towards competence as a GP and 'needs further development' is not a 'fail'.

- Give a 'competent' grade only when you are sure that the trainee's consultation deals adequately with the complexity within it and would clearly pass if it were a station at the CSA.

two assessments are often thought of as tools used in assessment *of* learning, but they are much more powerfully used in assessment *for* learning.)

Use of the COT and CbD is a way of holding up a mirror, so trainees can begin to see themselves and how they think and act. To make trainees effective self-directed learners, we need to encourage *metacognition* (making them aware of how they think). As the training period progresses, the trainer should regularly monitor signs that this journey towards self-directedness is taking place. If not, factors inhibiting progress must be searched for. They may include either learner or teacher factors.

Provision of choice in learning

Trainees are often anxious about knowledge and can put pressure on their trainer or consultant for teaching with high factual content or ask for time to read or go on courses that add to their knowledge. One of the aims of the GPStR training programme is to develop a level of tolerance for *not* knowing. It is not possible to 'complete' the GP curriculum in the three-year programme and know all there is to know about being a GP (indeed, would it ever be possible?). Instead we need to equip our trainees with insight into how to identify their areas for development and the skills to find things out safely.

Trainees should gradually be made more aware of two truths about general practice:

1 ◊ wisdom is usually more important than knowledge
2 ◊ we must accept some uncertainty as unavoidable; it pays to get used to not knowing.

Box 15.3 describes three ways of thinking about the role of the curriculum. We can see that in GP training we should be moving towards the second and third approach.

BOX 15.3 Ways of approaching the curriculum

1 □ Curriculum as a blueprint
Knowledge resides in the teacher and is transmitted. Education is a product. The teacher is implementing someone else's plan. The quality of learning depends on the teacher's performance. Assessment takes place at the end, and is mainly summative.

2 □ Curriculum as an aid
Knowledge is promoted. This sort of teacher is a facilitator who sets up learning opportunities. The learner is a seeker of knowledge. Assessment becomes part of teaching and is mainly formative.

3 □ Curriculum as a starting point
Interactivity. Both teacher and learner are explorers. This sort of teacher is a facilitator who learns alongside the learner. The important knowledge is understanding – the knowing that isn't in textbooks but discovered and created in interactions with patients, knowledge-in-action. Assessment is mainly self-assessment and this represents true self-directedness.

Source: from Fish and Coles (2005),[5] based on Habermas and Stenhouse.

At the same time, we should not underestimate the importance of factual knowledge in general practice. Trainers and clinical and educational supervisors need to maintain a strategic view that includes assessing both the quality of trainees' knowledge, and their ability to develop a mature and responsible self-directed attitude to evaluating their knowledge and filling gaps. Box 15.4 contains some suggestions for planning the content of the final year or training in practice, as an example of this progression.

BOX 15.4 Delivering content

First weeks in general practice
- Induction: building relationship and trust, familiarisation with practice systems.
- Patient safety, e.g. NICE referral guidelines for cancer.
- Focus on common condition the GPStR sees in surgery.
- Prioritise needed topics (e.g. what to take with you to an emergency visit, acute meningococcal infection) and areas that hold particular anxiety for the GPStR.

Middle of the attachment
- Concentrate on the basic competences that relate to the doctor–patient interaction: *primary care management, person-centred care and specific problem-solving skills.*
- Start to fill in content area blanks identified by e-portfolio.
- Address less common disorders that might not occur very frequently.
- Evidence-based treatment, e.g. Clinical Evidence, Bandolier, etc.

- Make the GPStR aware of NHS priorities (sometimes not identified as priority learning by trainees).

Later in the attachment
- Move onto the three advanced competences that move beyond the doctor–patient interaction: *a comprehensive approach, community orientation* and *a holistic approach.*

- Begin to deal with increasing complexity in diagnosis and management.

- Continue to fill in content area gaps identified by e-portfolio (and consider why they are gaps).

- After the CSA, address in greater depth non-clinical areas such as prevention, screening, professionalism, medico-legal, self-awareness (often such topics are not seen as priority learning).

159

Anchoring teaching on cases seen by the GPStR makes sure that topics are mapped closely to learners' needs. This is not to say that the cases seen by the trainee are typical of general practice as a whole (their case mix tends to differ in age and conditions presented). However, early in training, relating teaching almost exclusively to cases seen helps to keep the content of teaching close to perceived needs of the learner and is more satisfactory than planning lots of topic-based tutorials.

Content-free planning is where the teacher has a clear idea of the goal and the process but the content is provided by the learner: 'Planning involves thinking through what happened in the last lesson and getting a sense of direction and so it is then possible to wait for the task to emerge.'[6]

Box 15.5 is one example of how this can be done.

BOX 15.5 Example of how to plan teaching without knowing the topic

- Flexible lesson plans work best. Start with a clear idea about the overall goal of the session (what you want the trainee to come away with).

- Let the trainee tell the story of the case with as few interruptions as possible (only clarifying facts).

- Whilst listening, jot down possible areas for discussion (issues raised).

- Ask trainee to identify issues raised; get him or her to generate a list to encourage divergent and generic thinking.

- Deal with the trainee-identified issues first (can use or abandon your own list as you see fit).

- Encourage the trainee to identify decision points, analyse options and make judgements.

- Ask the trainee to summarise the discussion and say what he or she plans to do differently.

- Make a note of this change and *ask about it later* until he or she has achieved the change.

On-the-job and off-the-job learning

Honey and Mumford have represented the varied sources of learning and this is reproduced in Figure 15.2.

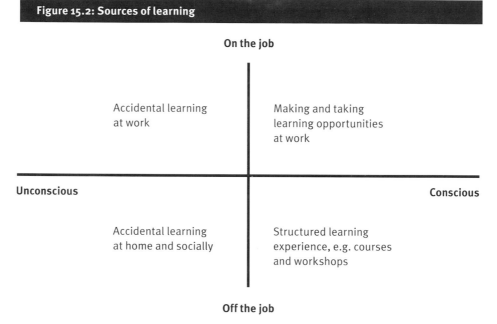

Figure 15.2: Sources of learning

On the job

Accidental learning at work

Making and taking learning opportunities at work

Unconscious — Conscious

Accidental learning at home and socially

Structured learning experience, e.g. courses and workshops

Off the job

Source: Mohanna, Wall and Chambers (2004).[7] Reproduced by permission of Radcliffe Publishing.

Educational providers will be thinking about all these sources of learning, taking the opportunity to redesign teaching and learning activities, and offering a varied diet of resources that can be flexible and responsive to learners' needs. Different modalities can be employed to address different types of content, learners with different learning styles and the preferences of teachers.

Small-group learning

The half-day release scheme in general practice vocational training has been described as the jewel in the crown of general practice education. Over the years these small-group learning opportunities have provided much-needed balance for the time spent training for general practice in hospitals.

Teaching through the new GP curriculum has the potential to build on this success, and incorporate a mix of activities for GPStRs at all stages of training. It might mean that the traditional half-day release from practice will not be available for all learners all the time and that a GPStR will need to take more personal responsibility for how his or her time is spent. In particular in

secondary care placements, specialty organised teaching, adapted for the needs
of those aiming to work in the community but run by secondary care teachers,
might be more appropriate. At other times, attendance will be key in gaining
those important skills of group membership and negotiation with others. Running
groups and sharing expertise, planning and facilitating sessions, team working
and problem-based learning are all activities that work well in the half-day
release setting. Expert educational supervision and an 'intelligent' PDP will
guide when each activity is appropriate for each GPStR.

   This style of learning prepares learners well for independent, lifelong learning.
Successful completion of the flexible GPStR programme should perhaps be best
seen as more important as preparation for professional life itself, rather than
just for entry into professional life.

Online learning

It is unrealistic to expect all learners to need the same things in terms of educational provision at the same time. Although all assessors are testing the same
things, the rate and stage at which learners need learning to help them deal
safely with practice will vary. Online resources can address this variation. They
are particularly effective for just-in-time-learning, providing solutions to problems in practice as they arise. Box 15.6 provides examples.

> **BOX 15.6 Online resources**
>
> **www.bmjlearning.com** □ a site run by the *British Medical Journal* (BMJ) editorial team
> aimed solely at online learning and recording of information. The site hosts a large
> number of learning modules, although you need to be a member of the British Medical
> Association (BMA) to access it for free.
>
> **www.doctors.net.uk** □ offers an email service and chat forums as well as online learning
> resources for most specialties, in addition to other elements such as medical news.
>
> **www.gpnotebook.co.uk** □ an excellent resource to use whilst in a consultation. The
> content is linked together in a very intuitive way that allows finding information easy.
> Primarily an online encyclopaedia of medical conditions, it also allows a PDP tracking
> facility.
>
> **www.onmedica.net** □ an online learning portal that provides a number of free resources
> primarily aimed at GPs. A PDP tracker tool is available that allows items read on the
> website (and other learning activities) to be recorded under the GMC PDP headings
> and also integrated into other applications such as the NHS Appraisal Toolkit. Features
> include articles, interactive courses and cases, journal round-up and a daily medico-
> political news service aimed at primary care.
>
> **The future**
> Where is all of this going in the future? Many sites offer two-way interactivity. Sites such
> as Wikipedia allow visitors to make changes to the sites themselves. The next generation

Continued over

162

of internet tools such as Internet Explorer 7, Office 2007 and Windows Vista will allow people to aggregate and customise the information they want to see. Many other sites that allow users to upload and flag popular content are now gaining in momentum, like YouTube (videos) and Flickr (photos), and there are networking sites such as Facebook.

So, we may soon have the ability to create our own mobile intranets using websites containing the information we use on a daily basis. Perhaps Primary Care Trusts may even start offering their information and guidance in the form of RSS feeds. (RSS stands for Really Simple Syndication and is a particular kind of web page specially for material that changes frequently and can be updated.) Could we see the National Institute for Health and Clinical Excellence offering a consultation document that clinicians can make comments upon and share in real time? Programme directors, educational supervisors and trainers can now think about putting together interactive local resources to support learning activities.

Source: adapted from a list compiled by Luke Koupparis, Medical Editor of www.onmedica.net, and reproduced with permission.

Summary

Responsibility for planning education lies with the learner and not with the trainer. The trainer should supervise progress and provide formative assessment to allow development of self-directedness. Educational providers need to make the most of the opportunity to provide a variety of activities and guide learners to choose and use resources appropriately. This approach to educational development links well with the model that we see in the NHS appraisal process. Although currently the e-portfolio and the NHS Toolkit are not compatible, maybe in the future this will be an area that will be developed. This will make appraisal and Personal Development Planning a natural extension of training.

REFERENCES

1. Stenhouse L. Some limitations of the use of objectives in curriculum research and planning *Paedagogica Europaea* 1970; 6: 73–83.

2. Kolb D A, Fry R. Toward an applied theory of experiential learning. In: C Cooper (ed.). *Theories of Group Process*, pp. 138–56, London: John Wiley, 1975.

3. Honey P, Mumford A. *Using Your Learning Styles* Maidenhead: Peter Honey, 1986.

4. Jennings S F. Personal development plans and self-directed learning for healthcare professionals: are they evidence based? *Postgraduate Medical Journal* 2007; 83(982): 518–24.

5. Fish D, Coles C. *Medical Education: developing a curriculum for practice* Maidenhead: Open University Press, 2005.

6. Brown L, Coles A. Complex decision-making in the classroom: the teacher as an intuitive practitioner. In: T Atkinson, G Claxton (eds). *The Intuitive Practitioner: on the value of not always knowing what one is doing*, pp. 165–81, Buckingham: Open University Press, 2000.

7. Mohanna K, Wall D, Chambers R. *Teaching Made Easy* (second edn) Oxford: Radcliffe Medical Press, 2004

Teaching about personal and professional responsibilities in the new curriculum

Mike Deighan

This chapter starts by exploring the complex nature of professionalism, which is seen differently by every author. This diversity of opinion poses problems for both teachers and learners. The chapter continues with a discussion of why professional responsibilities have recently become more important and controversial. The next area to be explored is equally problematic: how can professional responsibilities be taught? The chapter ends by dealing with the areas of professional responsibility that most affect trainees and their learning.

The most important publication for the trainee is the General Medical Council's *Good Medical Practice*,[1] which sets out our professional responsibilities in the section 'Duties of a Doctor' (see Box 16.1). However, although this document tells the trainee what to do and why the issues are important, it doesn't explain how professionalism should be learnt.

BOX 16.1 Duties of a doctor

Patients must be able to trust doctors with their lives and health. To justify that trust you must show respect for human life and you must:

- make the care of your patient your first concern

- protect and promote the health of patients and the public

- provide a good standard of practice and care:
  - keep your professional knowledge and skills up to date
  - recognise and work within the limits of your competence
  - work with colleagues in the ways that best serves patients' interests

- treat patients as individuals and respect their dignity:
  - treat patients politely and considerately
  - respect patients' right to confidentiality

- work in partnership with patients:
  - listen to patients and respond to their concerns and preferences
  - give patients the information they want or need in a way they can understand
  - respect patients' right to reach decisions with you about their treatment and care
  - support patients in caring for themselves to improve and maintain their health

---

Continued over

> - be honest and open, and act with integrity:
>   - ☐ act without delay if you have good reason to believe that you or a colleague may be putting patients at risk
>   - ☐ never discriminate unfairly against patients or colleagues
>   - ☐ never abuse your patients' trust in you or the public's trust in the profession.

164

The nature of professionalism

There is good agreement on the definition of *a profession*, the Royal College of Physicians (RCP) definition (see Box 16.2) being very similar to that of former Chief Medical Officer Sir Kenneth Calman[3] a decade before.

BOX 16.2 What is a profession?

The RCP definition[2]

- A profession is an occupation whose core element is work based upon the mastery of a complex body of knowledge and skills.

- It is a vocation in which knowledge of some department of science or learning, or the practice of an art founded upon it, is used in the service of others.

- Its members profess a commitment to competence, integrity and morality, altruism, and the promotion of the public good within their domain.

- These commitments form the basis of a social contract between a profession and society, which in return grants the profession the right to autonomy in practice and the privilege of self-regulation.

- Professions and their members are accountable to those served and to society.

Calman definition[3]

- It is a vocation or calling and implies service to others.

- It has a distinctive knowledge base that is kept up to date; it determines its own standards and sets its own examinations.

- It has a special relationship with those whom it serves – patients, clients.

- It has particular ethical principles – the ethical base.

- It is self-regulating and is accountable to patients and to the profession itself.

However, professionalism is less easily defined and is seen as 'a mixed bag' according to two key publications.[2,4]

Downie[5] simplifies things by identifying three themes within professionalism:

1 ◊ with patients and colleagues – *interpersonal professionalism*
2 ◊ as a profession – *public professionalism*
3 ◊ personal – *intrapersonal professionalism.*

This three-fold classification can be useful to learners in trying to make sense of the many strands of professionalism. Its possible use for teaching was explored by Van De Camp *et al.*[6] (see Table 16.1). What is remarkable about their study is the diversity of opinion about what is important.

TABLE 16.1 Aspects of professionalism

Interpersonal		Public (society)		Intrapersonal (self)	
Patients	Colleagues	Accountability	Quality	Personal qualities	Behaviours
Altruism	Relationships with colleagues	Submission to an ethical code	Use of explicit standards	Maturity	Lifelong learning
Tolerance	Interpersonal skills	Duty	Deliverance of quality	Humility	Good clinical judgement
Caring	Participation	High level of expertise	Commitment to excellence	Flexibility	Not letting personal beliefs influence care
Service	Asking for help when necessary	Professional conduct	Technical competence	Courage	Responding to stress
Responsibility	Teamwork	Calling	Adherence to guidelines	Motivation	Dealing with uncertainty
Compassion	Communication skills	Negotiation	Respecting expert authority	Humanistic values	Critical analysis
Politeness	Leadership	Justice	Transparency	Self-awareness	Knowing limits of professional
Integrity	Teaching colleagues	Method and thoroughness	Whistle-blowing if necessary	Temperance	Being well-organised
Honesty		Clear professional values			
Reliability		Enhancing the welfare of the community			
Avoiding misuse of power		Protect confidential information			

Continued over

Admitting errors in judgement	Commitment to continuity of patient care	-
Sensitivity to patient diversity	Commitment	
Educating patients		
Giving understandable information		
Respecting patients' right of shared decision making		
Setting appropriate limits		

Medicine and society: a social contract

A crisis in professionalism?

There are a number of potent social changes that are altering the nature of the relationship between doctor and patient (and between the medical profession and society). Some of them are listed by Stewart (see Box 16.3).

BOX 16.3 Changes in society affecting the doctor–patient partnership

- Rise of consumerism in medicine.
- Emphasis on patient autonomy.
- Changing status of women in society.
- The rise of a disabled culture of affirmative action and pride.
- Attacks on professional self-regulation.
- Increasingly litigious environment.
- Multiculturalism.
- Social concerns about assault and violence towards women.
- Holistic and alternative health movement.
- Change in status of all professions in society.
- Decline of role of medicine and expansion in role of other professionals.
- Increased use of technology.

- Shift of care from hospital to community.

- European working-time directive.

- Increased hospital liability for doctor's care.

- Administrative – containment of medical care costs.

- Increased emphasis on informed consent.

- Increased attention to prevention and patient education.

- Social acceptance of physician-assisted suicide.

- Doctor's role as trustee regarding disability benefits

Source: adapted from Stewart et al.[7]

The challenge in recent years to autonomy and accountability is one of the strongest drivers of change in the status of doctors, with the perception of many in society that the profession is arrogant and insensitive. It is acknowledged that the public's 'crisis of trust' goes beyond the medical profession (and we are still more trusted than politicians) but a loss of trust in doctors has been exacerbated by incidents such as Shipman, Bristol and Alder Hey.[8]

The profession's failure to convince the public about the merits of the measles, mumps and rubella immunisation (MMR) is a reminder of how dangerous (in terms of mortality and morbidity) a loss of trust can be. (For a summary of how this was reported in the media, see http://news.bbc.co.uk/1/hi/in_depth/health/2002/mmr_debate/default.stm.)

> Professional status is not an inherent right, but is granted by society. Its maintenance depends on the public's belief that professionals are trustworthy and to remain trustworthy, professionals must meet the obligations expected by society.[9]

Most people trust their doctors, but this does not mean the trust is well placed. For example, Illich[10] argued that modern medicine does more harm than good, partly through iatrogenic harm, but mainly by exercising political power and monopolising health care. A doctrine of 'experts know best' has undermined people's ability to deal with their own illness and heal themselves. Whilst these ideas are too radical for some commentators, it is important that learners are prepared to question assumptions and examine the claims of modern medicine in an open way. Like other professions,[11] doctors should question whether they can continue to view themselves as neutral within society.

Living in an imperfect world

Another problem for medicine and society to deal with is medical fallibility; Gawande points out that medicine[12] *is an imperfect science, an enterprise of constantly changing knowledge, uncertain information, fallible individuals and, at the same time, lives on the line. There is science in what we do ... but also habit, intuition, and sometimes plain old guessing. The gap between what we know and what we aim for persists. And this gap complicates everything that we do. ... As pervasive as medicine has become in modern life, it remains mostly hidden and often misunderstood. We have taken it to be both more perfect than it is and less extraordinary than it can be.*

Schön expands on this, pointing out the uncertain nature of professional decision making. How important this is, and how unrecognised by those who take a technical managerialist approach through risk management and clinical governance!

In the varied topography of professional practice, there is a high, hard ground overlooking a swamp. On the high ground, manageable problems lend themselves to solution through the application of research-based theory and technique. In the swampy lowland, messy, confusing problems defy technical solutions. The irony of this situation is that the problems of the high ground tend to be relatively unimportant to individuals or society at large, however great their technical interest may be, while in the swamp lie the problems of greatest human concern.[13]

These words seem to apply particularly to general practice, and there are implications for teaching. Sometimes trainees look to deal with things in the manageable, clear-cut way they have been familiar with, in 'high ground' surgical procedures or the technical medical world. They need to be led into the swamp. And they need teachers who both recognise the difference between the swamp and the high ground, and who can help with the uncertainties lurking there.

The struggle to stay centred on values

Each day, physicians fight to express values in the face of reality. This is referred to by Inui[4] who contrasts the ideal with the reality (see Table 16.2).

TABLE 16.2 **The struggle to stay centred on values in the profession of medicine**

Value	The ideal	The reality
Truth/science	Evidence-based	Uncertainty
Therapeutic alliance	Confluence of interest	Conflict of interest
Curing	Caring, healing	Risk, harming
Accepting, empathic	Open heart, open mind	Arrogant, unmoved
Right action	Error-free	Mistake-prone
Reflective	Analytic	Hassled, knee-jerk
Altruistic	Self-sacrificing	Avaricious

Learners need to be made aware of these struggles, to experience them for themselves and to reflect on them. They provide excellent material for case-based discussions.

Teaching professionalism

Before looking at ways of teaching professionalism, it is worth considering how learners' professional values develop before they reach us. We have all witnessed changes in learners as they pass through medical school and house jobs. Stewart[7] suggests that, in learning to be physicians, learners pass through three phases (see Table 16.3).

TABLE 16.3 Physicians' learning – the human dimension		
Technical competence in dealing with disease	Developing a professional identity	Learning to heal
Medical students, biological sciences	Clinical clerkship and hospital training	This phase takes at least five to ten years
Value system of the medical establishment: ■ the primary task of medicine is the recognition and treatment of disease ■ everything else is peripheral – communication, psychological, social, and environmental factors	Work as part of the clinical team Have responsibility for patient care Begin to feel like doctors Usually become comfortable with their strengths and limitations Develop a clearer sense of their professional roles	Physicians learn to be instruments of healing, accepting with humility and wisdom the power to heal bestowed upon them by their patients
Deterioration in ability to communicate effectively with patients	Refine their ability to appraise critically their own performance	This phase is not accomplished by all physicians

In some ways, GP training is the development of the final phase and repair of harm done in the first two phases. This third stage will continue through specialty training and beyond:

It is important to note that learning to be a healer continues after formal education is completed. The seeds are planted during the training period, but only grow and develop as physicians experience the power of the healing relationship in practice.[7]

It is not possible to 'teach' this transition; learners have to make their own journey. 'One cannot will oneself to "believe" until one understands. But understanding often will only arise from experience. So it is necessary first to allow the experience to happen.'[14]

The reason why some physicians never learn to heal is because they cannot make what Schön calls a *suspension of disbelief.* This requires the student to: 'willingly suspend his disbelief in utterances [of the teacher] that seem false or even absurd. ... Disbelief must be suspended until [the student] has access to the information on which to base a good decision.'[13]

Intuition

Much learning relating to professionalism is intuitive:

> *Much of the time, experienced professionals ... cannot explain what they are doing, or tell you what they know; and students cannot articulate their learning. Yet professional development and practice are often discussed as if conscious understanding and deliberation are of the essence.*[15]

Narratives and stories[16] can be used to help explore professional responsibilities:

> *Educators can ... help by raising awareness, exploring the value of intuition in decision making, sharing intuitive experiences with learners, recognising the contributions (yet inherent ambiguities) of evidence-based practice, setting learning in such a way that the process of decision making is emphasised, and encouraging a non-judgemental no-blame environment when, after a 'reasonable' course of action, things turn out to be other than expected.*[17]

Can professional values be taught?

This may seem to imply that you cannot teach professionalism, that it is something the learner has to acquire for him or herself and may never learn. On the contrary, we can help trainees develop professional competence, but we need to remember that teaching and learning are not causally related. In other words, learning does not always follow teaching. However, although the success of our teaching depends on the learner's willingness to learn, we can influence that willingness in a number of ways.

Professional competence has been defined by Epstein[18] as:

> *the habitual and judicious use of communication, knowledge, technical skills, clinical reasoning, emotions, values, and reflection in daily practice for the benefit of the individual and the community being served.*

Many trainers and educational supervisors would feel confident that they could motivate a learner to improve his or her performance in all of the above fields.

Approaches to teaching professionalism

Up until recently, professionalism might not have been perceived as something that needed teaching. Rather it was seen as something that would be learned subconsciously by modelling. Now, more active methods are thought to be required. Several approaches are available:

1 ◊ apprenticeship
2 ◊ theory
3 ◊ technique or skills-based approach
4 ◊ reflective practice.

Historically, each approach has been in vogue in professional education at some time. When teaching professional responsibilities I would suggest using a variety of approaches:

- apprenticeship, which depends heavily on modelling, is suitable for conveying attitudinal aspects of professionalism, such as caring, commitment, altruism, tolerance, service, compassion and integrity
- theory can be used for GMC advice and information on ethical codes
- technique or skills-based approach is needed to instil the habits of lifelong learning, or for learning how to give understandable information to patients
- reflective practice can be used to improve clinical judgement or self-awareness. It makes for deep learning but is least useful when the learner is very new and has few experiences to reflect on.

Some aspects of professionalism suit a mixture of approaches. For instance, dealing with inappropriate professional attitudes to fellow team members might be taught by example, by theory (e.g. 'Twelve strategies for effective communication and collaboration in medical teams'[19]) or by means of a reflective discussion.

Using the humanities to explore professionalism

Trainees often have had relatively few major life experiences. Vicarious experience of fictional or real accounts of sickness, death and other, more positive, life experiences can help the learner understand a wider variety of perspectives on life. Trainees should be encouraged to watch TV, see films, read books and go to the theatre; their reading and watching (and that of their trainer or clinical supervisor) are legitimate topics for discussion in training.

Using assessment to explore professional responsibility

Multi-source feedback (MSF) and the patient satisfaction questionnaire (PSQ) are ways of bringing out aspects of professionalism that may be blind spots for the learner. Although giving the feedback may de difficult, it is an opportunity for quality learning. Case-based discussion (CbD) can also be used to explore skills, knowledge and attitudes on professionalism. A sequence of CbDs could be used to focus on an area where the trainee needs to develop.

The annual review of competence progression may throw up major issues of professional responsibility if the trainee has problems. This process is not punitive: the emphasis is on offering opportunities to the learner to recognise his or her learning needs and seek help.

Changing nature of personal responsibility

Many teachers are aware of a different work ethic in their trainees from that which was common while they themselves were training. Change in attitudes (often characterised as a move from 'idealism' to 'cynicism') can cause friction between the learner and the practice. It should be acknowledged that things have changed as regards attitudes to work and a study on this[20] is summarised in Table 16.3.

TABLE 16.3 **Changes in attitudes to work**				
	Traditionalists	**Baby boomers**	**Generation X**	**Generation Y**
Born	Pre-1946	1947–67	1968–80	1981–95
Attitudes and values	Loyalty	Personal growth	Independence	Confident
	Sacrifice	Youthfulness	Pragmatism	Optimistic
	Honour	Equality	Results-driven	Civic-minded
	Compliance	Ambition	Flexible and adaptive	Innovative
	Patient	Collaboration	Resourceful	Diversity-focused
	Commitment to hierarchical leadership	Optimistic	Cynical?	Lifelong learners
		Value status		Education key to success
Work	Hard-working	Workaholic	Results-driven	Work–life balance
	Dedication	Accept stress	Mistrustful	
Goal	To build a legacy	To put their stamp on things	To maintain independence in all areas of their lives	To find work and create a life that has meaning

Source: adapted from Lyons *et al.*[20] and Roberts.[21]

Professionalism incorporates advocacy for patients. It includes caring for patients throughout their healthcare journey, ensuring that they are well managed within the healthcare system and that one does not completely abdicate responsibility when one's case moves outside a given specialty area. Or, indeed, when ongoing care threatens to breach a 'working-time directive'. This is especially important in handover of patients to other colleagues.

Hours of work are often a cause of disagreement between learners and supervisors, and this issue is an example of a change in professionalism. Today it is not considered unprofessional to leave work at a reasonable time. It is however unprofessional to put a patient at risk by leaving without proper handover arrangements. Today's young doctors seek a better work–life balance and are not going to accept an outmoded workaholic approach. They have a different attitude to professional responsibility that ought to be respected (and perhaps learnt from) by their more senior colleagues.

Resources for teaching on the central issues in professionalism

Attitudes to clinical governance and patient safety

Most of this is learnt by observation. Good theoretical insights can be found from the National Patient Safety Agency website (www.npsa.nhs.uk/health/resources) (e.g. 'Seven steps to patient safety' or the 'Significant event audit') or from articles in the *British Medical Journal* careers supplement.

Ethics and values

Teaching about ethical issues starts with recognising ethical issues when they arise. One way to raise awareness of this is with random case analysis focusing only on ethical issues, or by asking the trainee to keep an ethics diary for a week – noting down issues that made him or her stop and think.

One basic approach is simply to discuss the difference between a rule-based approach (e.g. *always tell the patient the full truth*) and a consequentialist approach to ethics (... *but what if the truth upsets them and makes them worse?*). Trainees will often have a preference for either rules or pragmatism; to become patient-centred, they need to develop an awareness of their own preferences on ethical issues.

The four ethical principles[21] are often used in teaching. The principles should be set in context (for examples of this, see Molyneux,[22] who advocates a '9-Rule' method for considering ethical problems, or Sandars[23] and the medico-legal context). The British Medical Association website is excellent for practical advice on ethics.

Promoting equality and valuing diversity

Good equality and diversity practice is best taught by modelling it in the workplace. There are also good online courses[24] to increase awareness. Partly, this is taught as an important area of professional and personal development, but there are also diversity employment issues that the trainee will benefit from knowing about.

174

Evidence-based health care

Some see a conflict between patient-centred care and evidence-based health care (EBHC). On the one hand, some doctors avoid EBHC because it lacks humanity, while, on the other, Armstrong[25] warns that patient-centredness can be used as a rhetorical device to preserve the autonomy of the doctor against a prevailing set of practice standards and managerial imperatives.

Professional responsibility dictates that doctors use the best evidence available for diagnosis and treatment, and at the same time use a comprehensive and holistic approach. Humanity is not just being sympathetic but doing the best that can be done for the patient.

We need to raise awareness in trainees about the 'evidence' that makes up much of EBHC. Ideally they will develop a healthy degree of scepticism about research that is quantitative, by pharmaceutical companies and done only in secondary care and 'adapted' for primary care.

NICE, Clinical Evidence, Bandolier, *Drug and Therapeutics Bulletin* and the *MeReC Bulletin* are better sources of evidence than pharmaceutical representative-sponsored lectures in practices and postgraduate centres.

Teaching, mentoring and clinical supervision

One of the best ways of learning is to teach; it can lead to greater retention. Opportunities often exist for a GP specialty registrar (GPStR) to teach medical students, foundation doctors and fellow specialty registrars, in the practice, in hospitals and on day-release courses. If opportunities do not exist, it is worth trying to create them. Box 16.4 contains examples that might form the basis of a discussion between learners at different stages.

Experienced GPStRs should also be encouraged to train to use the workplace assessment tools and perform these for more junior trainees. Online resources[26] can be useful for theory.

BOX 16.4 **Examples of professionalism issues suitable for discussion with a GPStR**

- A doctor doing an intimate examination without a chaperone.

- A patient asking for a sick note who doesn't seem to deserve one.

- A colleague who is showing evidence of underperformance.

- Breaches of confidence.

- Issues of capacity and consent in minors and people with learning difficulty.

- A doctor prescribing a drug for an unlicensed indication.

- Meetings between doctors and pharmaceutical companies' medical representatives.

- Patient autonomy: any place for benign paternalism?

REFERENCES

1. General Medical Council. *Good Medical Practice* London: GMC, 2006.

2. Royal College of Physicians of London. *Doctors in Society: medical professionalism in a changing world* London: RCP, 2005.

3. Calman K. The profession of medicine *British Medical Journal* 1994; 309(6962): 1140–3.

4. Inui TS. *A Flag in the Wind: educating for professionalism in medicine* Washington, DC: Association of American Medical Colleges, 2003.

5. Downie RS. Professions and professionalism *Journal of Philosophy of Education* 1990; 24(2): 147–59.

6. Van De Camp K, Vernooij-Dassen MJ, Grol RP, *et al.* How to conceptualize professionalism: a qualitative study *Medical Teacher* 2004; 26(8): 696–702.

7. Stewart M, Brown J, Freeman T (eds). *Patient-Centred Medicine: transforming the Clinical Method* (second edn) Oxford: Radcliffe Medical Press, 2003.

8. O'Neill O. *Trust and Transparency*. BBC Radio 4 Reith Lectures – A Question Of Trust 2002, www.bbc.co.uk/print/radio4/reith2002/lecture4.shtml [accessed December 2007].

9. Cruess SR, Cruess RL. Professionalism must be taught *British Medical Journal* 1997; 315(7123): 1674–7.

10. Illich I. *Medical Nemesis: the expropriation of health* London: Marion Boyars, 1975.

11. Popkewitz TS. *Critical Studies in Teacher Education: its folklore, theory and practice* London: Falmer Press, 1987.

12. Gawande A. *Complications: a surgeon's notes on an imperfect science* London: Profile Books Ltd, 2002.

13. Schön D. *Educating the Reflective Practitioner: towards a design for teaching and learning in the professions* San Francisco, CA: Jossey-Bass, 1987.

14. Waters M. Educating the reflective GP: Schön revisited *Education for Primary Care* 2004; 15: 631–4.

15. Atkinson T, Claxton G. *The Intuitive Practitioner: on the value of not always knowing what one is doing* Buckingham: Open University Press, 2000.

16. Eggly S, Brennan S, Wiese-Rometsch W. 'Once when I was on call … ': theory versus reality in training for professionalism *Academic Medicine* 2005; 80(4): 371–5.

17. Pitts J. Intuition, medical practice and education *Education for Primary Care* 2001; 12: 264–6.

18. Epstein R, Hundert E. Defining and assessing professional competence *Journal of the American Medical Association* 2002; 287: 226–35.

19. Rider E. Twelve strategies for effective communication and collaboration in medical teams *BMJ Career Focus* 2002; 325(7359): S45.

20. Lyons S, Duxbury L, Higgins C. An empirical assessment of generational differences in work-related values. In: D M Zinni (ed.). *Annual Conference of the Administrative Sciences Association of Canada* Toronto, Ontario, 2005.

21. Roberts T. Can professionalism in medicine survive in a changing world? UKCEA Conference, 2007, www.gpkss.ac.uk/ukcea2007/index.php [accessed December 2007].

22. Gillon R. Medical ethics: four principles plus attention to scope *British Medical Journal* 1994; 309(6948): 184–8.

23. Molyneux D. Teaching ethics to GP registrars on the day-release course: an evaluation *Education for Primary Care* 2001; 12: 379–86.

24. Sandars J E, Newson L. *MRCGP: approaching the modular examination* (second edn) Knutsford: PasTest, 2002.

25. Hetherton M, Caldwell J. *Equality and Diversity* (UKCEA online course), 2006, www.doctors.net.uk/ecme/wfrmOverview.aspx?groupid=82&moduleid=581 [login required].

26. Armstrong D. Clinical autonomy, individual and collective: the problem of changing doctors' behaviour *Social Science and Medicine* 2002; 55: 1771–7.

27. Wilkie V. *Teaching Junior Doctors in General Practice* (UKCEA online course), 2006, www.doctors.net.uk/ecme/wfrmOverview.aspx?groupid=46&moduleid=466 [login required].

176

The self-evaluation tool

The Staffordshire Evaluation of Teaching Styles

This short questionnaire, the Staffordshire Evaluation of Teaching Styles (SETS), will help you to find out about your preferred teaching styles.

Please rate how much you agree with each of the statements below on the five-point scale. Remember that the scores range from 1, not agreeing at all, through to 5, which is very strongly agreeing. So the more you agree, the higher the score. Once you have scored yourself, then you will be able to map out your preferred teaching styles using the scoring grid that follows and put these scores into the six teaching styles diagram (Figure A1).

	not agree at all			strongly agree	
Q1 ☐ I vary my approach depending on my audience	1	2	3	4	5
Q2 ☐ I am less comfortable giving straight presentations than teaching through games and exercises	1	2	3	4	5
Q3 ☐ I prefer to teach through games to relay learning	1	2	3	4	5
Q4 ☐ I like having external targets to determine the course of learning	1	2	3	4	5
Q5 ☐ I prefer teaching sessions that are self-contained with no follow-up	1	2	3	4	5
Q6 ☐ Props often detract from a talk	1	2	3	4	5
Q7 ☐ I am comfortable addressing large audiences	1	2	3	4	5
Q8 ☐ Preparation for my teaching focuses on me and my role	1	2	3	4	5
Q9 ☐ I am usually standing up when I teach	1	2	3	4	5
Q10 ☐ The best teaching sessions convey straight facts in a clear way	1	2	3	4	5
Q11 ☐ I avoid being distracted from running sessions the way I plan to run them	1	2	3	4	5
Q12 ☐ I am happy teaching general skills	1	2	3	4	5

Continued over

178

	not agree at all			strongly agree	
Q13 ☐ I put no value on being formally employed as a teacher	1	2	3	4	5
Q14 ☐ I dislike one-to-one teaching	1	2	3	4	5
Q15 ☐ I am consistent in delivery of a topic, whatever the audience	1	2	3	4	5
Q16 ☐ I like to give students the opportunity to explore how to learn	1	2	3	4	5
Q17 ☐ I have developed my own style as a teacher	1	2	3	4	5
Q18 ☐ I prefer one-to-one teaching	1	2	3	4	5
Q19 ☐ Eliciting emotions through role-play or drama is a valuable aspect of teaching	1	2	3	4	5
Q20 ☐ I am comfortable using humour in my teaching	1	2	3	4	5
Q21 ☐ I am rarely sitting down when with the students	1	2	3	4	5
Q22 ☐ It is important to me that my teaching is accredited by an official body	1	2	3	4	5
Q23 ☐ I am uncomfortable when I have multi-professional groups of learners to teach	1	2	3	4	5
Q24 ☐ I am at my best when organising my teaching to fit an external curriculum or organisational structure	1	2	3	4	5

The scoring grid for the Staffordshire Evaluation of Teaching Styles tool

Once you have filled in your own scores for all of the 24 questions on the SETS questionnaire, you will need to transfer the score for each question into the six teaching styles. The questions on the SETS questionnaire have been randomly allocated, so it is important that you assign the marks correctly to each teaching style.

Please fill in your score for each of the questions in the correct boxes and then add the columns up to obtain your score for each of the six teaching styles (out of a maximum of 20 marks).

Question	Style One	Style Two	Style Three	Style Four	Style Five	Style Six
Q1	Q1 =					
Q2		Q2 =				
Q3		Q3 =				
Q4			Q4 =			
Q5						Q5 =
Q6						Q6 =
Q7					Q7 =	
Q8			Q8 =			
Q9					Q9 =	
Q10				Q10 =		
Q11				Q11 =		
Q12	Q12 =					
Q13						Q13 =
Q14					Q14 =	
Q15				Q15 –		
Q16		Q16 =				
Q17	Q17 =					
Q18						Q18 =
Q19		Q19 =				
Q20	Q20 =					
Q21					Q21 =	
Q22			Q22 =			
Q23				Q23 =		
Q24			Q24 =			
Totals						

Next, please fill in your scores obtained from the chart totals above, into the six boxes against each of the teaching styles below:

Your Scores

STYLE ONE: THE ALL-ROUND FLEXIBLE AND ADAPTABLE TEACHER
This teacher can use lots of different skills, can teach both peers and juniors, and is very aware of the whole environment both in teaching and of the learners.

STYLE TWO: THE STUDENT-CENTRED, SENSITIVE TEACHER
This teacher is very student centred, teaches in small groups, with emotions to the fore, using role-play and drama, and is not comfortable doing straight presentations.

STYLE THREE: THE OFFICIAL CURRICULUM TEACHER
This teacher is very well prepared as a teacher, accredited, is very aware of and teaches to the formal curriculum, and follows external targets for teaching.

STYLE FOUR: THE STRAIGHT-FACTS, NO-NONSENSE TEACHER
This teacher likes to teach the clear facts, with straight talking, concentrating on specific skills, and much prefers not to be involved with multidisciplinary teaching and learning.

STYLE FIVE: THE BIG CONFERENCE TEACHER
This teacher likes nothing better than to stand up in front of a big audience. This teacher does not like sitting in groups or one-to-one teaching.

STYLE SIX: THE ONE-OFF TEACHER
This teacher likes to deliver small self-contained bits of teaching, on a one-to-one basis, with no props to help and no follow-up.

So now you have the scores out of 20 for your own self-evaluation of your preferred teaching styles. Now please go on to Figure A1.

The Staffordshire Hexagon: a diagrammatic representation of your preferred teaching styles

Please take the marks (out of 20) from the scoring grid and put a cross along each of the six axes to represent your score in each of the six teaching styles.

You may wish to join up the crosses to produce a shape of your own combination of styles.

FIGURE A1 **The Staffordshire Hexagon**

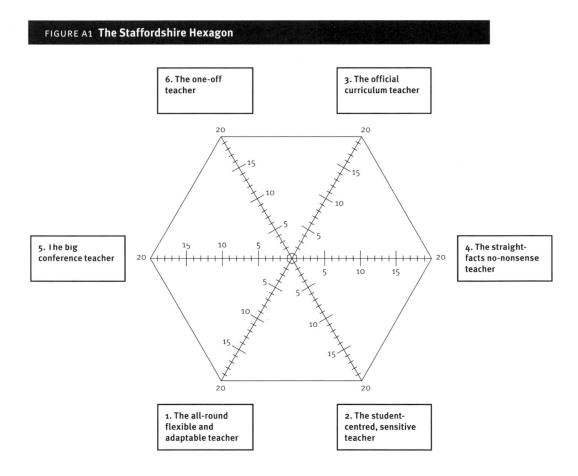

6. The one-off teacher

3. The official curriculum teacher

5. The big conference teacher

4. The straight-facts no-nonsense teacher

1. The all-round flexible and adaptable teacher

2. The student-centred, sensitive teacher

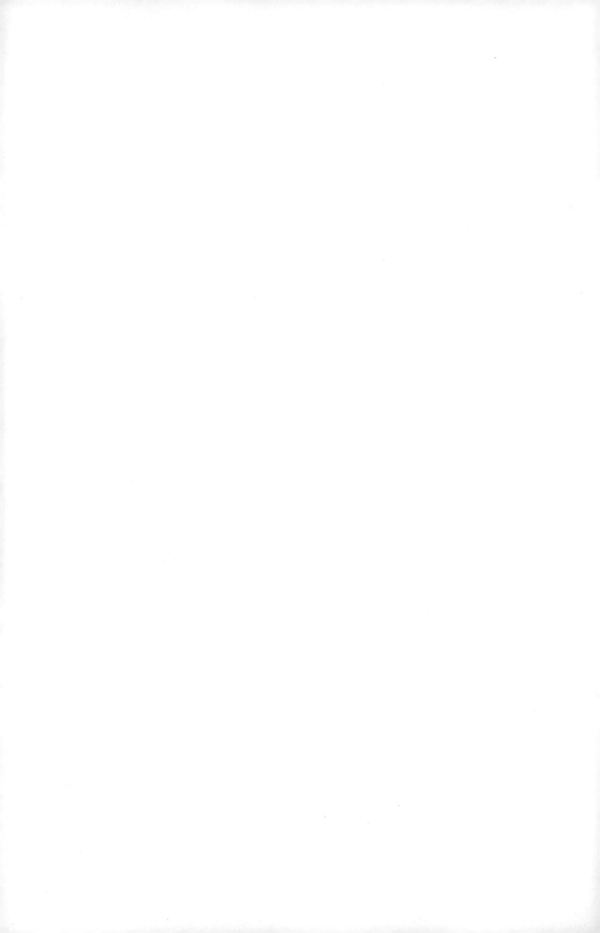

Index